NATIONAL ACADEMIES *Sciences Engineering Medicine*

NATIONAL ACADEMIES PRESS
Washington, DC

Optimizing Care Systems for People with Intellectual and Developmental Disabilities

Joe Alper, Rose Marie Martinez, and Kelly McHugh, *Rapporteurs*

Board on Population Health and Public Health Practice

Health and Medicine Division

Proceedings of a Workshop

THE NATIONAL ACADEMIES PRESS 500 Fifth Street, NW Washington, DC 20001

This activity was supported by an anonymous donor and the National Academies of Sciences, Engineering, and Medicine. Any opinions, findings, conclusions, or recommendations expressed in this publication do not necessarily reflect the views of any agency or organization that provided support for the project.

International Standard Book Number-13: 978-0-309-69060-7
International Standard Book Number-10: 0-309-69060-9
Digital Object Identifier: https://doi.org/10.17226/26624

This publication is available from the National Academies Press, 500 Fifth Street, NW, Keck 360, Washington, DC 20001; (800) 624-6242 or (202) 334-3313; http://www.nap.edu.

Copyright 2022 by the National Academy of Sciences. National Academies of Sciences, Engineering, and Medicine and National Academies Press and the graphical logos for each are all trademarks of the National Academy of Sciences. All rights reserved.

Printed in the United States of America.

Suggested citation: National Academies of Sciences, Engineering, and Medicine. 2022. *Optimizing care systems for people with intellectual and development disabilities: Proceedings of a workshop*. Washington, DC: The National Academies Press. https://doi.org/10.17226/26624.

The **National Academy of Sciences** was established in 1863 by an Act of Congress, signed by President Lincoln, as a private, nongovernmental institution to advise the nation on issues related to science and technology. Members are elected by their peers for outstanding contributions to research. Dr. Marcia McNutt is president.

The **National Academy of Engineering** was established in 1964 under the charter of the National Academy of Sciences to bring the practices of engineering to advising the nation. Members are elected by their peers for extraordinary contributions to engineering. Dr. John L. Anderson is president.

The **National Academy of Medicine** (formerly the Institute of Medicine) was established in 1970 under the charter of the National Academy of Sciences to advise the nation on medical and health issues. Members are elected by their peers for distinguished contributions to medicine and health. Dr. Victor J. Dzau is president.

The three Academies work together as the **National Academies of Sciences, Engineering, and Medicine** to provide independent, objective analysis and advice to the nation and conduct other activities to solve complex problems and inform public policy decisions. The Academies also encourage education and research, recognize outstanding contributions to knowledge, and increase public understanding in matters of science, engineering, and medicine.

Learn more about the National Academies of Sciences, Engineering, and Medicine at **www.nationalacademies.org**.

Consensus Study Reports published by the National Academies of Sciences, Engineering, and Medicine document the evidence-based consensus on the study's statement of task by an authoring committee of experts. Reports typically include findings, conclusions, and recommendations based on information gathered by the committee and the committee's deliberations. Each report has been subjected to a rigorous and independent peer-review process and it represents the position of the National Academies on the statement of task.

Proceedings published by the National Academies of Sciences, Engineering, and Medicine chronicle the presentations and discussions at a workshop, symposium, or other event convened by the National Academies. The statements and opinions contained in proceedings are those of the participants and are not endorsed by other participants, the planning committee, or the National Academies.

Rapid Expert Consultations published by the National Academies of Sciences, Engineering, and Medicine are authored by subject-matter experts on narrowly focused topics that can be supported by a body of evidence. The discussions contained in rapid expert consultations are considered those of the authors and do not contain policy recommendations. Rapid expert consultations are reviewed by the institution before release.

For information about other products and activities of the National Academies, please visit www.nationalacademies.org/about/whatwedo.

PLANNING COMMITTEE FOR A WORKSHOP ON OPTIMIZING CARE SYSTEMS FOR PEOPLE WITH INTELLECTUAL AND DEVELOPMENTAL DISABILITIES[1]

JAMES PERRIN (*Cochair*), John C. Robinson Chair in Pediatrics, Massachusetts General Hospital for Children, and Professor of Pediatrics, Harvard Medical School

HOANGMAI PHAM (*Cochair*), President, Institute for Exceptional Care

KARA AYERS, Assistant Professor of Pediatrics, University of Cincinnati College of Medicine

JULIA BASCOM, Executive Director, Autistic Self Advocacy Network

ALICIA THERESA FRANCESCA BAZZANO, Chief Health Officer, Special Olympics International

SUSAN THOMPSON HINGLE, Associate Dean, Center for Human and Organizational Potential, and Professor of Medicine at Southern Illinois University School of Medicine

ELIZABETH MAHAR, Director of Family and Sibling Initiatives at the Arc U.S.

SANDRA SCHNEIDER, Associate Executive Director, American College of Emergency Physicians

Health and Medicine Division Staff

ROSE MARIE MARTINEZ, Study Director and Senior Board Director, Board on Population Health and Public Health Practice

KELLY McHUGH, Research Associate

STEPHANIE HANSON, Research Associate (*until April 2022*)

DARA ROSENBERG, Research Associate

GRACE READING, Senior Program Assistant

Y. CRYSTI PARK, Administrative Assistant

Consultant

JOE ALPER, Consulting Writer

---

[1] The National Academies of Sciences, Engineering, and Medicine's planning committees are solely responsible for organizing the workshop, identifying topics, and choosing speakers. The responsibility for the published Proceedings of a Workshop rests with the workshop rapporteurs and the institution.

Reviewers

This Proceedings of a Workshop was reviewed in draft form by individuals chosen for their diverse perspectives and technical expertise. The purpose of this independent review is to provide candid and critical comments that will assist the National Academies of Sciences, Engineering, and Medicine in making each published proceedings as sound as possible and to ensure that it meets the institutional standards for quality, objectivity, evidence, and responsiveness to the charge. The review comments and draft manuscript remain confidential to protect the integrity of the process.

We thank the following individuals for their review of this proceedings:

DONNA M. FICK, Penn State College of Nursing
JANET SHOUSE, Vanderbilt Kennedy Center
MEGHAN WARREN, Patient-Centered Outcomes Research Institute

Although the reviewers listed above provided many constructive comments and suggestions, they were not asked to endorse the content of the proceedings nor did they see the final draft before its release. The review of this proceedings was overseen by **MAXINE HAYES,** School of Medicine, and School of Public Health, University of Washington. She was responsible for making certain that an independent examination of this proceedings was carried out in accordance with standards of the National Academies and that all review comments were carefully considered. Responsibility for the final content rests entirely with the rapporteurs and the National Academies.

Acknowledgments

The National Academies of Sciences, Engineering, and Medicine's Board on Population Health and Public Health Practice wishes to express its sincere gratitude to Planning Committee cochairs James Perrin and Hoangmai Pham for their valuable contributions to the development and orchestration of this workshop. The board also wishes to thank all the members of the planning committee and the staff who collaborated to ensure a workshop complete with informative presentations and rich discussions. Finally, the board thanks the speakers and moderators who generously shared their expertise and their time with workshop participants.

This activity was supported by an anonymous sponsor and the Board on Population Health and Public Health Practice of the National Academies of Sciences, Engineering, and Medicine.

Contents

ACRONYMS AND ABBREVIATIONS	xvii
PROCEEDINGS OF A WORKSHOP	1
DAY ONE: CURRENT CHALLENGES	1
INTRODUCTION	1
Conduct of the Workshop, 4	
ELEMENTS AND COMPETENCIES OF AN INTEGRATED SYSTEM OF CARE	5
Models of Care, 5	
Exploring Attitudes of Doctors Toward People with a Disability, 10	
Providing Hope, Support, and Information to Families, 13	
Discussion, 15	
CHALLENGES IN WORKFORCE STRENGTH AND PREPAREDNESS	16
Challenges Clinicians Face When Providing IDD Services, 17	
Barriers and Potential Solutions to Optimal Health Care for Patients with Disabilities, 20	
Challenges in Workforce Availability, Training, and Payment, 23	
Discussion, 25	
SPOTLIGHT PRESENTATION: OPERATION HOUSE CALL	25
CHALLENGES IN FINANCING AND PAYMENT	27
Challenges in Financing Payment for People with IDD, 27	
Measuring Quality in IDD Services, 30	

The Swiss Cheese of Financing Services and Supports for
    People with IDD, 32
Discussion, 33
CLOSING COMMENTS FOR DAY ONE   34
DAY TWO: CURRENT AND PROMISING INTERVENTIONS   36
INNOVATIVE MODELS OF CARE AND COORDINATION   36
    The CART Team, 36
    Healthy Option, Medical Excellence: The Huntsman Mental
        Health Institute Neurobehavior HOME Program, 39
    Optimizing Care Systems for People with IDD, 42
    Discussion, 44
SPOTLIGHT PRESENTATION: BUILDING A BEHAVIORAL
THERAPY METAVERSE   45
INNOVATIONS IN WORKFORCE SOLUTIONS: THE
ROLE OF GENERAL HEALTH CARE PROVIDERS   46
    ECHO Autism Communities, 46
    Medical Student Education, 49
    Partnering to Transform Health Outcomes for Persons
        with IDD, 51
    Discussion, 53
INNOVATIONS IN FINANCING AND PAYMENT   55
    Innovations in Payment and Financing for IDD Services, 55
    Person-Driven Outcomes, 58
    Innovative Value-Based Contracting and Alternative
        Payment Models, 61
    Discussion, 62
CLOSING COMMENTS FOR DAY TWO   63
DAY THREE: LOOKING FORWARD   64
CONSIDERING A NEW VISION FOR MODELS OF CARE   64
    Elements of System Transformation, 64
    Rethinking Holistic Coordination, Connections, and
        Integration for People with IDD, 67
    North Carolina's Integrated Care for Kids Model, 71
    Discussion, 73
SPOTLIGHT PRESENTATION: SPECIALIZED
TELEMEDICINE FOR INDIVIDUALS WITH IDD   74
TECHNICAL AND POLICY OPPORTUNITIES IN
FINANCING AND PAYMENT   74
    Risk Adjustment for Payment of Health and HCBS, 75
    Financing Care Systems for People with IDD, 77
    A Population Health Framework for Caring for Individuals
        with IDD, 78
    Discussion, 79

SCALING WORKFORCE SOLUTIONS	80
The Role of Professional Organizations in Moving the Field Forward, 81	
Disrupting the Systemic Barriers and Biases That Limit Options for Individuals with IDD, 82	
Potential Federal Policy Opportunities, 84	
Discussion, 86	
CLOSING COMMENTS DAY THREE	88
REFERENCES	91
APPENDIX A: WORKSHOP AGENDA	95
APPENDIX B: STATEMENT OF TASK	99
APPENDIX C: BIOGRAPHICAL SKETCHES OF THE SPEAKERS AND MODERATORS	101

Box, Figures, and Tables

BOX

1 A working list of holistic coordinated functions, 68

FIGURES

1 The services that families and children with special health care needs use, 7
2 A care map drawn by a patient and their family, 8
3 Essential capacities of IDD practices, 9
4 Core components of care systems for individuals with IDD, 10
5 Actions systems could take to improve care for people with IDD, 11
6 Historical life expectancy of individuals with IDD, 17
7 Number of people living in a given setting by size, 1980–2030 (estimated), 18
8 Public spending on IDD services, 1977–2015, 19
9 NCQA's LTSS quality framework, 59

TABLES

1 Strategies to Address the Holes in Financing Services and Supports for Individuals with IDD, 33
2 NCQA's Proposed Person-Driven Outcome Measures, 60

Acronyms and Abbreviations

AAMC	Association of American Medical Colleges
ADA	Americans with Disabilities Act
AMA	American Medical Association
CCA	Commonwealth Care Alliance
CDC	Centers for Disease Control and Prevention
CHIP	Children's Health Insurance Program
CMMI	Center for Medicaid & Medicare Innovation
CMS	Centers for Medicare & Medicaid Services
COVID-19	coronavirus disease 2019
DD Act	Developmental Disabilities Assistance and Bill of Rights Act
DPC	Domestic Policy Council
DSP	direct support professional
ECHO	Extension for Community Healthcare Outcomes
ED	emergency department
EPSDT	early and periodic screening, diagnostic, and treatment
F2F	family-to-family
FQHC	federally qualified health center
HCBS	home and community-based services
HHS	Department of Health and Human Services

HOME	Healthy Options, Medical Excellence
HUD	Department of Housing and Urban Development
ICF/ID	intermediate care facilities for individuals with intellectual disability
IDD	intellectual and developmental disability
LCME	Liaison Committee on Medical Education
LTSS	long-term services and supports
NBS	Newborn Screening
NCD	National Council on Disability
NCQA	National Committee for Quality Assurance
PATH	Partnering to Transform Health Outcomes with Persons with IDD
PWIDD	persons with IDD

PROCEEDINGS OF A WORKSHOP

DAY ONE: CURRENT CHALLENGES

INTRODUCTION[1]

Approximately 7.4 million people in the United States[2] live with an intellectual or developmental disability (IDD) (Larson et al., 2001). According to a report from the U.S. Surgeon General (U.S. Public Health Service, 2001), individuals with IDD face exceptional challenges to staying healthy and getting appropriate health services when they are sick. Though the nation has taken important steps in the two decades since the release of that report, people with IDD still face significant barriers that impede greater access to quality health care and meeting their health goals. These barriers include being excluded from public campaigns to promote wellness, difficulty finding health care professionals who will accept them as patients and know how to meet their specialized needs, and struggling with unwieldy payment structures designed when people with IDD often died young or spent their lives in residential institutions (NCD, 2009).

---

[1] The planning committee's role was limited to planning the workshop, and the Proceedings of a Workshop was prepared by the workshop rapporteurs as a factual summary of what occurred at the workshop. Statements, recommendations, and opinions expressed are those of individual presenters and participants, and are not necessarily endorsed or verified by the National Academies of Sciences, Engineering, and Medicine, and they should not be construed as reflecting any group consensus.

[2] Available at https://publications.ici.umn.edu/risp/2017/infographics/people-with-idd-in-the-united-states-and-the-proportion-who-receive-services (accessed April 28, 2022).

IDDs are usually present at birth and negatively affect the trajectory of physical, intellectual, and/or emotional development;[3] many affect multiple body parts or systems. The Centers for Disease Control and Prevention (CDC) defines developmental disabilities as "a group of conditions due to an impairment in physical, learning, language, or behavior areas. These conditions begin during the developmental period, may impact day-to-day functioning, and usually last throughout a person's lifetime."[4] The American Association on Intellectual and Developmental Disabilities defines an intellectual disability as "a disability characterized by significant limitations in both intellectual functioning and in adaptive behavior, which covers many everyday social and practical skills. This disability originates before the age of 22."[5]

To explore the challenges and opportunities for creating an optimal care system for individuals with IDD, the National Academies of Sciences, Engineering, and Medicine (the National Academies) Board on Population Health and Public Health Practice hosted a three-part virtual public workshop, Optimizing Care Systems for People with Intellectual and Developmental Disabilities, on December 8, 10, and 14, 2021. It featured invited presentations and discussions that explored questions related to models of care, workforce, cross-discipline and cross-sector coordination, and financing and payment for care, such as the following:

- Models of Care
    - What are illustrative examples of care models that deliver holistic, tailored, developmentally appropriate, patient-centered, and coordinated care?
    - What factors limit the sustainability and/or adoption of these care models?
- Workforce Issues
    - What is known about the workforce that serves people with IDD?
    - What are the facilitators and barriers to improving the competency and capacity of all clinicians to care for people with IDD, particularly those individuals from minority and poor populations?
- Financing of and Payment for Care
    - What key data and analytic gaps do payers and purchasers need addressed to design effective financing and payment approaches for IDD care?

---

[3] Developmental Disabilities Assistance and Bill of Rights Act of 2000, Public Law 402, 106th Congress, 2nd session (October 30, 2000).

[4] Available at https://www.cdc.gov/ncbddd/developmentaldisabilities/facts.html (accessed April 28, 2022).

[5] Available at https://www.aaidd.org/intellectual-disability/definition (accessed April 28, 2022).

- What policy or programmatic changes would be required to ensure appropriate levels of financing for IDD health care services, including support for clinical providers to coordinate with peers in other service domains?

In her introductory remarks, Kimberly Knackstedt, Director of Disability Policy for the White House Domestic Policy Council (DPC), explained that DPC's role is to advise the president on policy across all domestic issues, with four teams focused on health and veterans, economic mobility, immigration, and racial justice and equity. The latter team, which Knackstedt belongs to, coordinates closely with the other teams to ensure equity is embedded in all policy development and action across the federal government. Knackstedt noted that her role of focusing on policies related to disability is new under the Biden administration, with prior administrations focused primarily on outreach regarding disability. "We now coordinate on outreach and work to embed disability policy into the president's agenda," she said. "This is so important because it is how we got to where we are today with disability priorities in the American Rescue Plan, the infrastructure bill, and at the forefront of the Build Back Better Act."

Knackstedt pointed out that the COVID-19 pandemic has laid bare inequities in the U.S. health care system and highlighted the long-term care crisis in the nation, in terms of both the lack of a sufficient workforce and the infrastructure and system deficiencies that adversely affect service delivery. She noted that while many individuals with disabilities prefer to receive care in their homes, delivery of home- and community-based services also faces challenges. "We have a shortage of home help and direct support workers, a limited supply of accessible, affordable housing, and difficulties accessing home and community-based services," she said.

During the 2020 presidential campaign, candidate Biden committed to working to ensure that people with disabilities have the choices and opportunities to fully participate in the community. "That was not a false promise, and in nearly a year, we have already seen that promise take shape in several ways," said Knackstedt. The American Rescue Plan,[6] for example, makes a significant down payment in the form of billions of dollars in additional Medicaid funding for 1 year to support an infrastructure for home-based caregiving

---

[6] The president signed into law H.R. 1319, the American Rescue Plan Act of 2021 on March 11, 2021. The law provides additional relief to address the continued impact of the COVID-19 pandemic on the economy, public health, state and local governments, individuals, and businesses. https://www.whitehouse.gov/briefing-room/legislation/2021/03/11/bill-signing-h-r-1319 (accessed April 28, 2022).

and community-based services. This investment has helped expand access to services and ensure that caregivers receive fair compensation for their work.

The administration is also prioritizing community living through interagency collaboration, such as the partnership between the Departments of Health and Human Services (HHS) and Housing and Urban Development (HUD). This collaboration, announced in July 2021, should increase access to accessible and affordable housing and the services that support community living for people with disabilities and older adults. HHS and HUD are also working to strengthen partnerships between housing and service networks at state and local levels to streamline access to both housing and community services for people with disabilities.

The takeaway, said Knackstedt, is that the Biden administration is committed to a significant, long-term investment in the U.S. caregiving infrastructure. The Build Back Better Act, for example, was passed on November 19, 2021, and included funds that will reduce waitlists for the more than 800,000 people who need home care. It will permanently improve Medicaid coverage for home care services, making community living a reality for thousands, and improve the quality of caregiving jobs, through not only the Medicaid proposal but a separate proposal that supports recruitment, training, and retention to support caregivers, which would improve the quality of care.

Knackstedt pointed out that policy makers are listening to the IDD community's concerns and working to make changes and improvements to the care system. She added that all of this work is grounded in equity, both from the administrative side and in its work with Congress on the legislative agenda. "The president's primary goal is to ensure that all Americans, including people with disabilities, live in a society that is accessible, inclusive, and equitable," said Knackstedt. "We are working to ensure that disabled Americans are at the forefront of our policy development and deeply embedded into how we think and act when implementing our goals."

She said that while the COVID-19 pandemic stressed the U.S. care infrastructure as never before, the nation is on the brink of a monumental shift to support people with disabilities living independently and accessing services and supporting caregivers. "We are finally at a moment to look forward, find hope, and most importantly, to build back better together," said Knackstedt.

Conduct of the Workshop

An ad hoc planning committee organized the 3-day virtual workshop (see Appendix A for the agenda) in accordance with National Academies procedures. The planning committee members were Kara Ayers, Julia Bascom, Alicia Theresa Francesca Bazzano, Susan Thompson Hingle, Elizabeth Mahar, James Perrin (cochair), Hoangmai Pham (cochair), and Sandra Schneider. The workshop was broadcast live over the web, and workshop presentations were posted to the web along with links to the videos of the talks.[7] Appendixes B and C contain the Statement of Task and biographical sketches of the speakers and moderators, respectively.

This publication summarizes the workshop's presentations and discussions. In accordance with National Academies policies, the workshop did not attempt to establish any conclusions or recommendations about needs and future directions, focusing instead on issues identified by individual speakers and participants. The summary was drafted by rapporteur Joe Alper in collaboration with National Academies staff members Rose Marie Martinez, Kelly McHugh, and Y. Crysti Park as a factual account of what occurred, and the National Academies does not endorse or verify the statements.

ELEMENTS AND COMPETENCIES OF AN INTEGRATED SYSTEM OF CARE

The first session aimed to provide a framing and foundation for the rest of the presentations and discussions by explaining what subsequent sessions would mean when discussing care systems and what the most important features of an ideal care system would be. The session's three speakers were Edward Schor (Stanford University),[8] Lisa Iezzoni (Harvard Medical School), and Nanfi N. Lubogo (PATH CT and Family Voices). James Perrin (Massachusetts General Hospital for Children and Harvard Medical School) moderated a discussion following the three presentations.

Models of Care

Not long ago, people with IDD, along with people with serious emotional disorders and various neurologic conditions, spent much of their lives in asylums, said Schor. These institutions were considered places of shelter and support; however, many provided poor living conditions and little treatment and were felt to violate human rights. Beginning in the 1950s and continuing for several decades, public institutions for individuals with IDD closed, with

---

[7] Available at https://www.nationalacademies.org/event/12-08-2021/exploring-an-optimal-integrated-care-system-for-people-with-intellectual-and-developmental-disabilities-a-workshop-day-1; https://www.nationalacademies.org/event/12-10-2021/exploring-an-optimal-integrated-care-system-for-people-with-intellectual-and-developmental-disabilities-a-workshop-day-2; and https://www.nationalacademies.org/event/12-14-2021/exploring-an-optimal-integrated-care-system-for-people-with-intellectual-and-developmental-disabilities-a-workshop-day-3 (accessed April 28, 2022).

[8] Complete affiliation and titles are available in the speaker biographical sketches in Appendix B.

the intent of replacing them with comprehensive, high-quality, community-based services and care. "Unfortunately, in many ways, we continue to wait for that best practice model of service to be available," said Schor.

Abundant research documents the failures of the current U.S. health care system, said Schor. These failures have created problems for everyone who uses health care, which are particularly apparent and consequential for individuals who have special care needs, including those with IDD. Generic problems with the U.S. health care system that affect people with IDD include significant disparities in access and quality of health services that affect health status, dissatisfaction with care expressed by both patients and caregivers, and unreliable quality of care that is often substandard compared to people without disabilities. Driving these problems, said Schor, is that clinicians and health systems fail to understand the special needs of people with IDD; design care to align with the special needs, goals, and priorities of people with IDD; and recognize their limited capacity in terms of professional skills to address these special needs.

Though the structure and operation of health care systems play a critical role in how care is provided to those with IDD, they and their families also rely on many other systems, given that almost no individual with IDD has only cognitive or developmental challenges (see Figure 1). "Consequently, for their needs be met well, they require access to multiple systems of services and supports that, in the best of all worlds, share goals and coordinate care," said Schor. The ideal care system would integrate all of these services, but in the short term, it would be good if these services were at least well coordinated, meaning that patient care activities are deliberately organized and the providers readily and regularly share information. However, the reality is that care generally is not well coordinated, either among health care providers or across sectors. As a result, responsibility for care coordination typically falls to the patients and their families.

Good care for people with IDD must start with a care plan, he said, particularly because their care depends on multiple disciplines and services. Developing that plan starts with a comprehensive assessment that identifies issues affecting an individual's health and use of health care services and also involves the patient and their family or caregivers in partnership with their service providers setting treatment goals and priorities, identifying the actions needed to achieve those goals, and assigning accountability for each of those actions. Documenting the resulting care plan in writing and sharing it with the entire team of people and programs involved with serving the individual is essential for this process to work, said Schor.

One way to start assessing needs is to ask the patient and family to draw a care map that documents the multiple services they already use (see Figure 2). One thing Schor has learned from reviewing a group of care maps

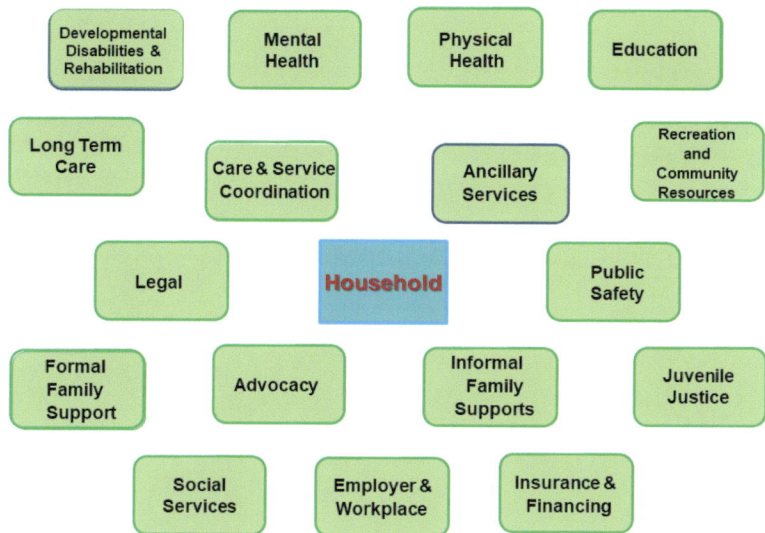

FIGURE 1 The services that families and children with special health care needs use.
SOURCES: As presented by Edward Schor at the workshop on Optimizing Care Systems for People with Intellectual and Developmental Disabilities on December 8, 2021; Schor slide 4 (data from Schor, 2019).

that families created for their children with special health care needs is that emotional support was the service listed most consistently, followed by health insurance and the services that medical specialists, primary care practices, and schools provide.

In many ways, said Schor, the service needs of people with IDD and their families are like those of other individuals with chronic health conditions. Individuals with IDD tend to be high users of health care services, particularly emergency departments (EDs) and neurologic, orthopedic, ophthalmologic, and psychiatric or behavioral services. Still, many individuals with IDD have unmet needs. In addition to depending on many other service sectors, perhaps what is most special about their needs is a desire for care that is sensitive, empathic, and able to account for their communication difficulties. Moreover, patients and caregivers consistently report feeling socially isolated, which can affect adherence to care plans and aggravate emotional and behavioral problems.

Getting necessary and appropriate care in the U.S. health care system can be demanding for anyone, but obtaining and coordinating it for people with IDD can be especially burdensome for their caregivers, who report a great deal of physical and psychological stress. However, said Schor, their burdens are not

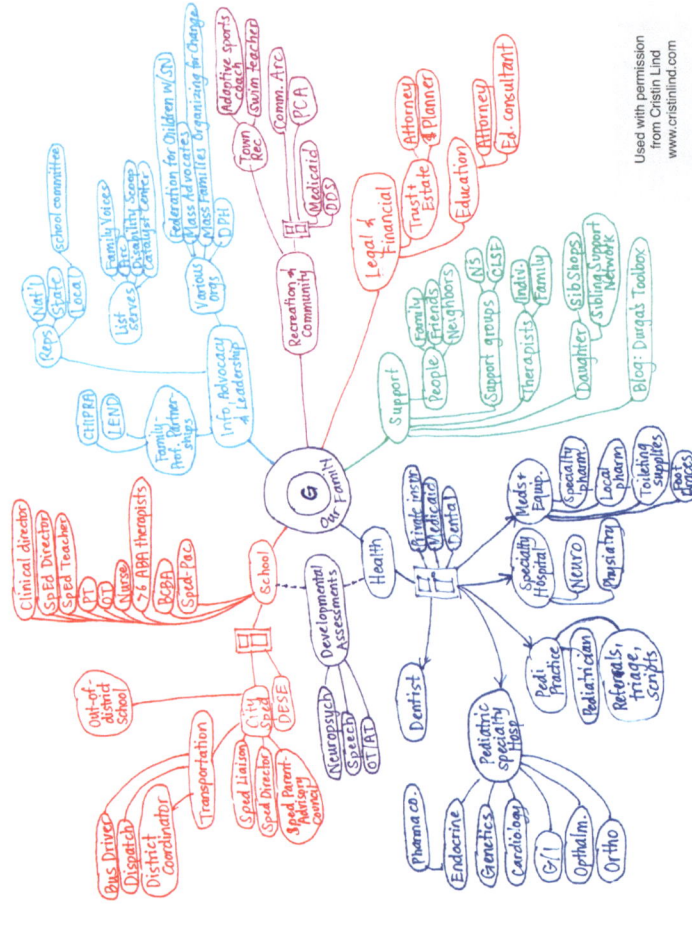

FIGURE 2 A care map drawn by a patient and their family.
SOURCES: As presented by Edward Schor at the workshop on Optimizing Care Systems for People with Intellectual and Developmental Disabilities on December 8, 2021; Cristin Lind, www.cristinlind.com.

solely or even primarily the result of care needs but most often the fault of the systems on which they depend. Caregivers often experience these systems as being inaccessible, unresponsive, uninformed, fragmented, and poorly coordinated. Often complicating matters, Schor added, is that patients with IDD and their families are more susceptible to adverse circumstances created by the communities they live in, which can aggravate health conditions or impede access to appropriate, equitable care.

Schor identified a consensus that good-quality care begins with access to a medical practice that provides care conforming to the medical home concept. In that model, a multidisciplinary team provides care that is patient and family centered, community based, comprehensive, coordinated, accessible, compassionate, continuous, and developmentally, cognitively, and culturally effective. Figure 3 lists the essential capacities that practices serving individuals with IDD should include (Sullivan et al., 2018).

Schor pointed out the important differences between the training and orientation of health care providers serving children versus adults. The differences in the experience of care in each setting can create difficult transitions from pediatric to adult health care for young adults with IDD. He noted that a group in Canada has developed an excellent set of clinical guidelines for primary care practices caring for adults with IDD (Sullivan et al., 2018), most of which apply to children with IDD. He added that the chronic care model (Bodenheimer et al., 2002) outlines a care model that can guide system design to meet the needs of this special population.

He listed a compilation of components and characteristics that a broad array of stakeholders has deemed essential attributes of systems caring for people with chronic conditions (see Figure 4). "This is an aspirational but achievable list that health care reform efforts should be addressing," said

- Assessment-based care planning & monitoring
- Life course health care and transition planning
- Functional assessment
- Adequate time
- Peer and family support
- Medication management
- Individualized, primary contact in the practice
- Technology: telehealth, electronic medical records
- Linkages to and coordination with frequently used resources, programs, social and mental health services
- Linkages Individual patient advocacy, e.g., participation in an Individualized Education Program
- Continuous quality improvement

FIGURE 3 Essential capacities of IDD practices.
SOURCES: As presented by Edward Schor at the workshop on Optimizing Care Systems for People with Intellectual and Developmental Disabilities on December 8, 2021; Schor slide 8 (data from Sullivan et al., 2018).

- Screen for eligibility and do outreach for enrollment
- Equitable access to assessment-based, comprehensive, evidence-based care
- Medical home certification for primary care practices
- Adequate, trained primary care and referral network
- Patient-professional partnerships at the system and practice levels
- Planned and facilitated transition from pediatric to adult care
- Health information technology to support individual care and population health
- Well-defined metrics for ongoing quality assurance & improvement
- Insurance & financing to minimize family financial burden and maintain needed benefits
- Adequate payment for team-base care, care coordination, dental and mental health services
- Whole family care including addressing social determinants of health and family quality of life

FIGURE 4 Core components of care systems for individuals with IDD.
SOURCE: As presented by Edward Schor at the workshop on Optimizing Care Systems for People with Intellectual and Developmental Disabilities on December 8, 2021; Schor slide 9.

Schor. Health care payers and health plans create policies that set the parameters for practices, he explained. Directly and indirectly, those parameters determine how practices organize and staff themselves and what services they offer. Whether benefits and coverage are adequate for people with IDD and whether practices can provide necessary care depends on whether these systems incorporate policies to ensure access to good-quality care for all individuals, especially those with special health care needs.

Many barriers exist to creating effective systems for people with IDD, but drawing on their and their families' expertise and the strength of the multiple interdependent system sectors on which they depend can overcome many of these, said Schor. As a starting point, he listed actions to improve care that the Agency for Healthcare Research and Quality has identified (see Figure 5) (AHRQ, 2014). "While these activities are not intended specifically to improve systems serving people with IDD, they offer a good starting place toward achieving that goal," Schor said.

Exploring Attitudes of Doctors Toward People with Disability, Including Intellectual Disability

To start her presentation, Lisa Iezzoni asked why, when the Americans with Disabilities Act (ADA) was passed over 30 years ago, people with disabilities still confront barriers and experience disparities in their health care in 2021. Surveys, focus groups, and in-depth interviews with people with a disability have identified a number of potential causes for these disparities:

- Measure performance and provide feedback to practices
- Transparent quality reports including achievement of patient-specific goals
- Support education and technical assistance to improve care for special populations
- Incentivize medical home certification
- Prevent secondary disabilities and promote well-being of patients and families
- Provide adequate payment for comprehensive, coordinated care
- Underwrite the costs of adopting health information technologies
- Foster systemwide adoption of best practices

FIGURE 5 Actions systems could take to improve care for people with IDD.
SOURCES: As presented by Edward Schor at the workshop on Optimizing Care Systems for People with Intellectual and Developmental Disabilities on December 8, 2021; Schor slide 10 (data from AHRQ, 2014).

- Complex underlying health conditions may require more attention than routine tests, such as mammograms.
- People with disability are often poor, have low education, and have problems with housing, food, transportation, and other essential services.
- Doctors receive inadequate training on and knowledge about disabilities, leading them to provide inadequate care for people with disability.
- Medical equipment such as exam tables is often inaccessible for people with a disability.
- Doctors, like much of society, make erroneous assumptions about and have discriminatory attitudes about people with disabilities.

Iezzoni and her collaborators conducted the first national survey about doctors' experiences with and perceptions about caring for people with a disability (Iezzoni et al., 2021). To develop the survey, her team conducted in-depth individual interviews with 20 practicing doctors in Massachusetts and three focus groups with 22 practicing doctors across 17 states. After testing the survey using eight cognitive interviews and pilot tests—the final survey had eight modules with 75 questions—they surveyed 1,400 physicians across 7 specialties (internal medicine, family practice, rheumatology, neurology, ophthalmology, orthopedic surgery, and obstetrics and gynecology). They included a $50 bill with the mailed survey as an inducement to participate; the response rate was 61 percent.

Eighty-two percent of respondents reported that people with significant disability have worse quality of life overall compared with other people. Only 41 percent reported they were strongly confident in their ability to provide equal-quality care to people with a disability, and 56 percent strongly welcomed people with disability into their practices. Doctors who finished medical school less than 20 years ago were more likely to report treating people with IDD. Responding to a question about the broader health care system, 21 and 47 percent, respectively, said that people with IDD had much worse or a little worse quality of care than other people.

Regarding communication, 70 percent of primary care physicians and 85 percent of specialists said they usually or always communicated with someone other than the individual with IDD. Among White doctors, 73 percent always or usually communicated with someone else compared to 83 percent of doctors who identified as belonging to a racial or ethnic minority. Responding to survey questions about whether they ever sedated individuals with significant IDD to perform routine, office-based tests or treatments, 8 percent of male physicians and 8 percent of primary care physicians said yes, compared to 18 percent of female physicians and 18 percent of specialists. Over twice as many rural doctors compared to urban doctors said yes to performing sedation—22 percent versus 10 percent—as did 14 percent of physicians who saw five or fewer individuals with an intellectual disability a month compared to 5 percent of those who saw six or more.

Iezzoni indicated that the survey had limitations: it was short, broad but shallow, and lacking questions that explicitly linked doctors' attitudes with their treatment decisions. In addition, budgetary concerns limited the survey size, so her team could not compare findings across specialties and the survey could not include other relevant specialties, such as pediatrics.

The issue of reproductive health for people with intellectual disability was a common theme that arose during the initial interviews and focus groups conducted to inform survey design. "There were some appalling things said by doctors whose expressions did not change when they said these things, so obviously they felt completely okay about saying these things," said Iezzoni. As an example, she recounted one comment she heard: "These patients are sexually active, and so contraception when they come to see me that is the real issue…. People who cooperate, we put in IUDs … I medicate as best as I can…. For those who don't cooperate, there is Depo-Provera and sterilization as needed."

Iezzoni reiterated that 82 percent of physicians said that people with significant disability have worse quality of life. This response raises questions about care for people with disability in times of scarce resources, such as during the COVID-19 pandemic. Given the potential bias that response uncovers, Iezzoni wondered whether it is possible to ensure that people with disability can get equal quality of care. "Why should patients with disability need to prove to their doctor that they value the quality of their life to get equal quality of care?" she asked.

Providing Hope, Support, and Information to Families

Nanfi Lubogo opened her presentation by explaining that Family Voices is a national organization and grassroots network of families and friends of children and youth with special health care needs and disabilities. The organization promotes partnerships with families, including those of cultural, linguistic, and geographic diversity, to improve health care services and policies for children (Family Voices, n.d.). Through its leadership in family-professional partnerships, Family Voices serves as the National Assistance Center for family-led centers funded by the Network of Maternal and Child Health. The 59 family-to-family (F2F) health information centers in all states, U.S. territories, and tribal nations have provided support and services to over one million families.

Lubogo said that Family Voices serves children who are at increased risk for chronic, physical, developmental, behavioral, or emotional conditions and need health and health-related services beyond those that children generally require. The organization also supports individuals with IDD affected by severe chronic conditions resulting from mental or physical impairments, who typically require long-term care for daily activities, such as mobility, health care, self-care, and independent living. Of the children and youth with special health care needs, Lubogo noted that 68 percent have two or more health conditions, 45.5 percent have health conditions affecting their daily lives, and 37.5 percent require specialized medical care. In addition, 32.2 percent require mental health care and 47.2 percent have needed mental or behavioral health care but did not receive it.

The COVID-19 pandemic made life extremely difficult for families of children with special health care needs or of individuals with IDD. Many were completely isolated for months and lost access to health care services or received fewer hours of in-home and/or skilled nursing supports. Lubogo's family lost in-home support services provided by the Department of Developmental Services for their 22-year-old daughter, who had just graduated from her post-high-school transition program.

That isolation affected her daughter's mental health, which took a turn for the worse during the pandemic. When she had a crisis, Lubogo could not get her an in-office appointment, and nobody would prescribe medication without first seeing her. When Lubogo called Connecticut's social needs help line, she was told to take her daughter to the ED, but the ED said no one could accompany her daughter, which was not a good option because she needed her family's support. Lubogo and her husband chose to ride out the storm at home and deal with their daughter's issues for almost 2.5 months until their mental health providers were able to use Telehealth to change her medication and provide therapy.

Through the Coronavirus Aid, Relief, and Economic Security (CARES) Act of 2020, Family Voices received $1 million and was able to provide telehealth technical assistance to the F2F centers, with 26 centers purchasing equipment to increase families' access to telehealth, 30 purchasing equipment to increase staff capacity, and 17 expanding hours or contracting with a cultural liaison to increase services to underserved communities. Thirty-five F2F centers developed new partnerships with Title V programs, state agencies, family-led community-based organizations, federally qualified health centers (FQHC), American Academy of Pediatrics chapters, and regional genetics networks to increase telehealth services. Lubogo noted that once these partnerships formed, families and the organizations involved began pushing to get families engaged in talking to health care providers about how to offer appropriate services for their children.

To participate in program design and identify priority areas, Family Voices developed the family engagement in systems assessment tool.[9] This tool promotes meaningful engagement of families in creating and improving policies, practices, and services. As an example, Lubogo recalled when the Connecticut Newborn Diagnosis & Treatment Network (Newborn Screening [NBS] program) approached her organization for help creating a family advisory group comprising families whose children were flagged during the screening process for a genetic condition. The NBS program also wanted help improving the screening process, identifying gaps in screening and diagnosis, and providing training and facilitation for staff so they can understand the needs of these families. Using their tool, Lubogo and her colleagues were able to identify priority areas, measure meaningful engagement with families, and conduct quality improvement strategies as needed.

Engaging families in health systems is a challenge, said Lubogo. The data resource center of the Child and Adolescent Health Measurement Initiative reported that 85.6 percent of children do not receive care in well-functioning systems, such as medical homes. During the COVID-19 pandemic, youth ages 18 and older were struggling with the transition to adult health care services. The data resource center also found that health care systems did not adequately involve families as equal partners. Other challenges included inequitable access to telehealth services, particularly for non-English speakers who could not access translation services during a telehealth visit and for families and individuals with IDD who were deaf or hard of hearing. In addition, some communities did not use telehealth at all, preferring to communicate using other technologies, such as the WhatsApp mobile phone application.

To ensure equity in all aspects of health care delivery, Lubogo and her colleagues are training providers about the effects of systemic racism on their

---

[9] Additional information is available at https://familyvoices.org/fesat.

care of individuals with intersecting marginalized identities, such as race, disability, and gender. They are also engaging families in co-designing health care programs, telehealth services, and policies, as well as coordinating care across subspecialties and systems, particularly for youth with special health care needs and IDD. Family Voices created an anti-racism initiative "Family Voices United to End Racism of Children and Youth with Special Health Care Needs and Their Families," launched on November 30, 2021, with 130 attendees from family organizations, Title V organizations, and managed care organizations. This initiative has held eight town halls and disseminated 12 resource documents to support further learning related to racism, segregation, and schools; mental health; the juvenile justice system and school-to-prison pipeline, health, Black culture and "the Talk," a discussion that Black families have with their children to teach them how to stay safe and survive encounters with the police.

Discussion

Perrin opened the discussion by asking the panelists how they would distinguish between what care systems should look like for adults versus children. From his perspective as a pediatrician, Schor said the place to start is to use pediatric practice as the baseline for designing adult practices because they have characteristics that adult practices should emulate. Pediatricians, for example, tend to talk to both the patient and family and spend more face-to-face time with their patients. Pediatrics also approaches prevention differently, creating more individualized approaches. Adult practices tend to follow the U.S. Preventive Services Task Force list of services rather than thinking about all the life-course implications of interventions.

Schor noted that both pediatric and adult practices are starting to colocate people, such as behavioral services and social services providers, and this would be a good feature to include in a practice model. Lubogo agreed that adult practices should model themselves after pediatric practices that serve as medical homes. She offered that collaboration and communication are necessary between pediatric and adult practices to prepare the adult practices for what they are going to face in transitioning to a better model of providing care.

Perrin then asked if adults and children with IDD get access to habilitative and rehabilitative services as part of home-based care; Iezzoni said it depends on the payer. She asked the other two panelists if they knew what happens when parents or other family caregivers become too functionally limited to provide in-home supports for an adult child. The key, said Schor, is to have relationships with other service providers so when that time comes, the adult caregivers can call on these connections. He added that during the pandemic, parents caught COVID-19 and did not have a backup for their child.

Lubogo noted that the most challenging time of transition occurs after age 26, when these children are considered real adults, by which time parents and families may be burned out or experiencing their own physical or mental health issues resulting from providing nonstop care for their loved ones. She hopes the federal government will provide more care for caregivers.

Iezzoni offered that her hope is that the next generation of physicians will be more enlightened than her generation. However, when a colleague of hers conducted implicit bias testing of medical students relating to disability, findings suggested high levels of implicit bias. She mentioned some research showing that the more time physicians spend with people with a disability, the more they realize that they are like other people. "I think that to the extent that we can encourage physicians—maybe through a continuing medical education requirement—to spend more time just getting to know people with disability outside of the care context, they will realize that they have a fine quality of life and that they often participate actively in their communities," she said.

Lubogo commented that this bias against individuals with a disability is systemic and societal, and the answer is to educate, educate, educate. One program, Operation House Call, has been training medical students in Connecticut and Massachusetts to identify their implicit biases and understand how these affect their care. She also suggested that working on equity and health equity would help address biases, whether about disability, race, or other marginalized traits.

As a final comment, Perrin wondered if the typical practice was capable of providing high-quality care to individuals with IDD. He believes the answer is no, which points to the need for better training. "The prevalence of IDD in the community is far greater than the prevalence of many of the conditions that medical students and residents learn how to manage," said Perrin, "so, there is a real failure to align training with what we know about the epidemiology of conditions in the general population, and there is also a great reluctance to change that training." Rather than creating specialized practices for people with IDD, training all physicians will be the most feasible approach to changing the status quo.

CHALLENGES IN WORKFORCE STRENGTH AND PREPAREDNESS

The second session featured three panelists who addressed the gaps in workforce capabilities and preparedness: Matt Holder (American Academy of Developmental Medicine and Dentistry), Susan Havercamp (The Ohio State University), and Amy Hewitt (University of Minnesota, Institute on Community Integration). Kara Ayers (University of Cincinnati College of Medicine) moderated the session and discussion period.

Challenges Clinicians Face in Providing IDD Services

Clinicians face six major challenges in caring for individuals with IDD, said Holder:

- inadequate professional knowledge and experience;
- patient complexity and the additional time it takes to assess and treat people who are complex in their presentations;
- diagnostic overshadowing;[10] which leads to
- overuse and polypharmacy;
- office modifications and training required by ADA; and
- improper reimbursement mechanisms.

He noted that the last challenge appears to be the most difficult one, but when it is solved, many of the other challenges are addressed as well.

Holder pointed out that until about 100 years ago, individuals with IDD were a pediatric concern because their life-spans were not long enough to result in a substantial adult population. When their life-spans began to increase (see Figure 6), the institutional system, which is where most young adults with IDD would live, became segregated from society.

It was not until the late 1990s, said Holder, that the nation prioritized keeping people with IDD living in the community (see Figure 7), and then

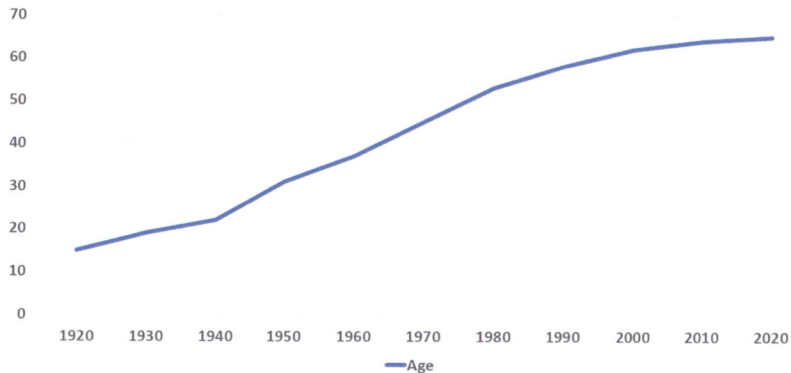

FIGURE 6 Historical life expectancy of individuals with IDD.
SOURCE: As presented by Matt Holder at the workshop on Optimizing Care Systems for People with Intellectual and Developmental Disabilities on December 8, 2021; Holder slide 4.

---

[10] Diagnostic overshadowing occurs when an individuals' health needs are frequently interpreted only in reference to their disability and not in regards to broader issues.

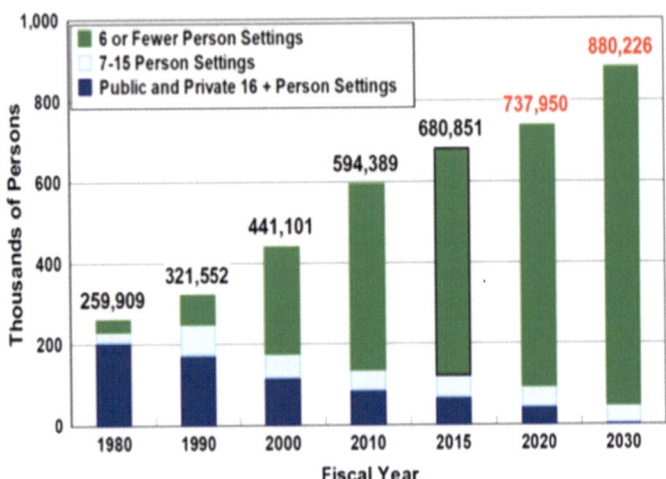

FIGURE 7 Number of people living in a given setting by size, 1980–2030 (estimated).
SOURCES: As presented by Matt Holder at the workshop on Optimizing Care Systems for People with Intellectual and Developmental Disabilities on December 8, 2021; Holder slide 5 (Lulinski et al., 2018).

spending on community care exceeded that for institutional care (see Figure 8) (Lulinski et al., 2018). One negative of this transition was that the expertise of the clinicians who worked in those institutions and spent every day and every patient encounter with a person with IDD was lost. "Suddenly, we had this large influx into the community of people who were older and had developmental disabilities, and there was this assumption that the clinicians who were out there would be ready, willing, and able to provide good care," said Holder. "That was not the case."

A 2002 report from the Surgeon General, *Closing the Gap*, detailed the known problems and gaps in providing care for individuals with IDD. Holder said the two main points were that provider education and payment were big problems. Not long after, the American Academy of Developmental Medicine and Dentistry came into existence; one of its first activities was to survey medical students and family medicine and internal medicine residency programs to quantify the training problem. It found that 81 percent of medical students, 85 percent of family medicine residents, and 95 percent of internal medicine residents received no clinical training about treating an adult with IDD. Those who did spent an average of 11 minutes on the subject.

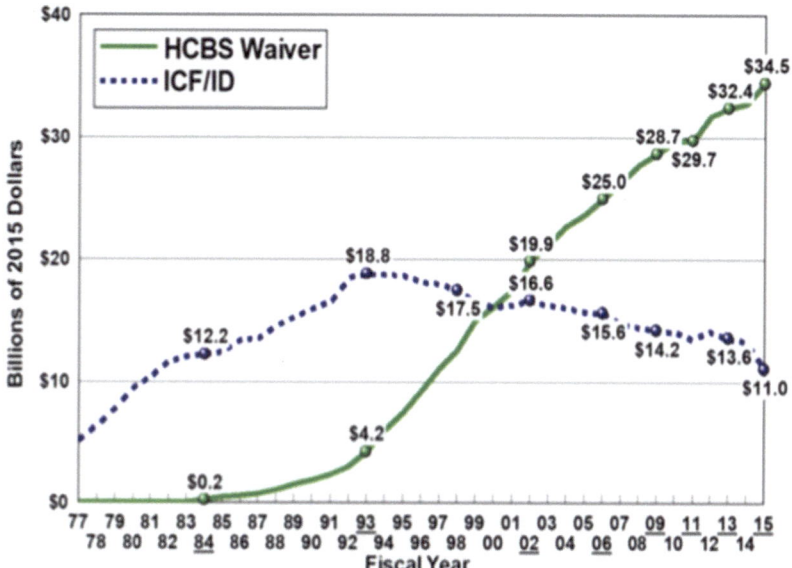

FIGURE 8 Public spending on IDD services, 1977–2015.
NOTE: HCBS: home and community-based services; ICF/ID: intermediate care facilities for individuals with intellectual disability.
SOURCES: As presented by Matt Holder at the workshop on Optimizing Care Systems for People with Intellectual and Developmental Disabilities on December 8, 2021; Holder slide 5 (Lulinski et al., 2018).

The sheer diversity of the genetic syndromes that include neurodevelopmental disorders makes physicians uncomfortable, said Holder. Roughly 1,000 named neurodevelopmental disorders exist, and the affected individuals show up at a medical practices with seizure disorders, intellectual disability, autism, psychiatric disorders, neuromuscular issues, communication difficulties, and all types of overlapping and overlaying issues that make assessment complex. He recalled that his organization had a large database at one time of physicians, dentists, physical therapists, and optometrists nationwide who had come to its events and were interested in working with this population. These clinicians did not necessarily have much training, but they were willing. However, as they gained some knowledge, they encountered a higher level of complexity with which they were uncomfortable.

What this illustrates, said Holder, is that access to care does not guarantee quality of care. "We can start with solving the access problem, but there is a level of complexity that we have to acknowledge and we have to plan around," he said. This level of complexity turns into diagnostic overshadowing (physicians blame a new medical or behavioral problem on an existing disability).

For example, an individual with Down syndrome may experience a decline in mental functioning that a physician might dismiss as something that happens to those with Down syndrome and fail to investigate other medical causes, such as a thyroid disorder.

Clinicians experienced in caring for individuals with IDD observe a classic cycle in some of their colleagues. It starts with a behavior complaint related to constipation, for example. The treatment is a laxative, but because of the individual's behavior, they receive an antipsychotic agent or benzodiazepine instead, which does nothing to treat constipation, which then gets worse. If the only way an individual has to communicate is through behavior, that behavior is going to worsen, which completes the cycle.

The end result of diagnostic overshadowing is overprescribing and polypharmacy that addresses the wrong problem. Almost half of the psychotropic drugs and 13 percent of anti-seizure drugs prescribed to individuals with IDD lack a corresponding diagnosis. "That is pretty shocking to me, and it should be to anybody who is thinking about quality of care," said Holder.

Turning to the challenge of inadequate reimbursement, Holder said that the clinic he runs gets only 25 percent of the reimbursement needed to provide the necessary quality of care. "We are not just missing the mark by a little in terms of our reimbursement structures. We are missing the mark by a lot, and this is something that we have to focus on and address because this really gets in the way of everything else," said Holder. The problem arises because the mix of people with IDD that come to his specialty clinic, for example, skews toward those with more complex needs compared to the mix of those with IDD in the general population.

Barriers and Potential Solutions to Optimal Health Care for Patients with Disabilities

It is a simple fact, said Havercamp, that people with disabilities cannot get health care, so they get sick and die when they should not (ICS, 2016). Compared to peers without disabilities, adults with IDD are five, three, and two times more likely to have diabetes, arthritis, or cardiovascular disease or asthma, respectively (Reichard et al., 2011). These conditions, she said, are not related to or caused by disability and can be prevented or mitigated with quality health care (Krahn et al., 2006).

People with IDD experience environmental barriers to healthy behaviors and barriers to quality health care, including barriers at the health care system, clinical practice, and provider levels. Focusing on the latter, Havercamp said she hears from individuals with IDD that it is difficult for them to find a provider who is willing to care for them (WHO, 2011). As Holder pointed out, health care providers feel unprepared and uncomfortable caring for patients with disabilities, and would much rather refer them to a specialist (Wilkinson et al., 2012), despite the lack of a specialty or subspecialty specific to adults with IDD. Even when they do find a provider, individuals with disabilities say they feel ignored or unheard, rushed, and as if their concerns were not truly respected (Breslin and Yee, 2009).

As Iezzoni's research has shown, health care providers without training tend to severely underestimate the capabilities of people with disabilities, their health, and their quality of life (Iezzoni at al., 2021). They hold negative and inaccurate assumptions about their current functional status and what could be possible in the future for people with disabilities, said Havercamp. Health care providers focus on the disability and completely overlook other cultural, economic, and social determinants of health. In fact, she added, referring back to Holder's earlier comments on diagnostic overshadowing, health care providers tend to overlook health issues that do not have anything to do with the disability. "A patient may come in because of an earache, and the health care provider wants to ask them about when they started using a wheelchair or the origin of their disability," said Havercamp. In addition, a concern that she hears repeatedly from people with disabilities is that if there is anyone else in the room, the health care provider is far more likely to speak to that person instead.

In thinking about the pathways to creating a disability-competent workforce, Havercamp and her colleagues proposed a list of steps toward improving health care (Bowen et al., 2020):

1. Collectively decide what health care providers need to understand about disability.
2. Change training and licensure requirements to ensure disability training.
3. Develop evidence-based curricular elements to convey disability competencies.
4. Develop robust protocols to evaluate disability training.
5. Evaluate the impact of disability training on health care delivery and on health outcomes.
6. Explore health care delivery models/incentive structures to promote disability-competent care.

Regarding the first item, she noted that perhaps a couple dozen health educators are committed to training on disability and have developed wonderful, innovative curricula in medical, nursing, and allied health fields.

In her view, the first objective or milestone for building a disability-competent workforce is to agree on what health care professionals need to learn. The Alliance for Disability in Health Care Education developed a list of learning objectives; with CDC funding, Havercamp and her colleagues recruited a large group of stakeholders to review the list and identify what was missing, unclear, and inapplicable. Through an iterative Delphi process, the group arrived at a consensus that the learning objectives reflected the skills, attitudes, and behaviors that all health professionals need to deliver quality health care for individuals with IDD and other disabilities (Havercamp et al., 2021).

In addition to reviewing the learning objectives, disability stakeholders contributed to a list of guiding principles and core values for those who care for individuals with IDD. They said that health care professionals need to understand that people with disabilities are a demographic group that frequently uses the health care system but has trouble accessing quality services. In collaboration with disability stakeholders, Havercamp's team developed a set of guiding principles and six core competencies that define the standard for health care professional training (ADHCE, 2019; Havercamp et al., 2021):

1. Develop a contextual and conceptual framework on disabilities to understand disability in the context of health conditions and the individual's environment.
2. Develop professionalism and patient-centered care skills that go beyond what medical and nursing students are learning.
3. Understand the legal obligations and responsibilities that health professionals have to accommodate disability and treat that as a civil right.
4. Understand how to work as a member of a professional team and apply systems-based practice principles.
5. Develop specific skills in clinical assessment.
6. Learn how to provide clinical care over the life-span and during transitions.

Health care educators can use these core competencies to develop curricula, she noted.

To mitigate the bias against people with disabilities, it is essential to include them in the training process, said Havercamp. At her institution, students report that training that includes people with disabilities increased their understanding and made them feel more comfortable interacting with them (Crane et al., 2021). Havercamp said that she and her colleagues believe that disability content should be required for health care accreditation and for licensure. "We need to evaluate disability competence on board exams and other critical milestones for students and health care professionals, and we need to do some policy work to make this all stick," she said.

Challenges in Workforce Availability, Training, and Payment

Over the past 30 years, the evolution of community living for people with IDD has led to most of them living in their family home and not receiving any services from their state's developmental disability systems providers, said Hewitt. She also noted that the definition of community living has changed over that time from one that considered it to be any context but a large, state-run institution to a view that people with IDD are not only living in but belong in their communities. At the same time, the definition of an institution has changed from one where hundreds of people lived to any type of congregate care setting.

A peak population of nearly 200,000 people with IDD in institutional settings in the mid-1960s has declined to just under 18,000. Expenditures have also increased, with Medicaid spending growing from $15.7 billion in 1987 to $55.3 billion in 2017 as the number of people receiving Medicaid-funded HCBS has grown from 22,869 in 1987 to 860,500 in 2017. More importantly, said Hewitt, the quality of life for people with IDD has improved over that period. They have love, they work, they have homes of their own, they have fun, and they are integrated into their faith communities in ways that were once unimaginable, Hewitt emphasized.

A key factor that has helped make this change possible has been the services of direct support professionals (DSPs). Their profession is largely unknown, however, so their work lives, profession, and wages or ability to access affordable benefits have not improved over the past 30 years. Hewitt said that when adjusted for inflation, their wages have shrunk, as have training and professional development requirements, with no federally required trainings and little opportunity for advancement. Burnout has been ever present, and turnover rates have hovered around 50 percent. Vacancy rates are high, and employers, including families or individuals who hire their own employees, are having difficulty finding, recruiting, and retaining DSPs.

This workforce is the backbone of community living supports for people with IDD, and the system relies on them to ensure quality of care, said Hewitt. It supports the work that physicians and therapists do in the clinic, and DSPs play a critical role in ensuring that people with IDD have good nutrition, exercise, and other supports that influence health and wellness. However, the challenges this workforce faces, and the resulting shortage of DSPs, is leading to low quality of services and poor outcomes for people who depend on their services.

This is not a new problem, said Hewitt, but it has intensified over the past 30 years. "What makes things worse is that we know what the solutions are, we just have not had the political will and the social will in our communities to make the changes we need," she said. As a result, reputable organizations are now asking states to increase the size of the residential sites they can offer, and many providers are planning on closing group homes and employment programs, at least temporarily, because they cannot hire enough DSPs.

Hewitt describes the workforce as comprising interdisciplinary professionals who need an eclectic skill set. They have to be able to instruct people with IDD to gain new skills and provide treatments and administer medications, which are similar to many nursing skills. In fact, said Hewitt, DSPs do many things that many states do not allow licensed practical nurses to do. They spend time counseling, advising, and helping people with IDD make the best decisions for themselves, and they are often the professionals who engage in daily routine physical, occupational, and speech therapy.

One problem, said Hewitt, is that the Bureau of Labor Statistics does not have an occupational code for DSPs. She noted that they are different from home health aides, who come into a person's home and help with housekeeping, cooking, and other activities; personal care aides or personal care assistants, who come into a person's home and support them with activities of daily living, such as bathing, dressing, and grooming; or certified nursing assistants, who typically work in a nursing facility and help with positioning, lifting, transferring, toileting, and similar activities. "Direct support professionals are all of those things, but there are other competencies we expect them to have," said Hewitt. "We know what those competencies are, we just do not require training around them."

Despite good data on occupational titles that the Bureau of Labor Statistics tracks, such as personal care aides, however, lacking an occupational code, the number of DSPs is only estimated. Given the number of people who receive certain types of IDD-related care and knowing what staffing ratios are, Hewitt estimates approximately 1.3–1.4 million DSPs in the United States. The number of all direct care workers, which includes home care workers, residential care aids, nursing assistants in nursing homes, and DSPs, is approximately 4.5 million people, Hewitt said.

The projected job openings for direct care positions through 2028 was 8.2 million people before the COVID-19 pandemic hit, with the demand for these positions growing even more since, said Hewitt. Approximately 87 percent of DSPs are women, with an average age of 45–54, which suggests that a retirement wave could worsen the shortage even more. About 73 percent have formal education beyond high school. They are clearly essential workers, and Hewitt and her colleagues advocated during the early stages of the pandemic to get states to recognize them as such, something they did accomplish.

To provide a perspective on how the pandemic has made the situation worse, Hewitt noted that about 19 percent of DSPs reported a COVID-19 diagnosis, and another 8 percent said they experienced the symptoms but were never formally diagnosed. When asked about their own health and wellness as a result of the pandemic, 50 percent reported physical or emotional burnout, 47 percent high anxiety, 38 percent sleep difficulties, 18 percent health complications, and

4 percent suicidal ideation. "The pandemic has affected this workforce in some real and challenging ways, and their work-life balance is getting much, much more difficult for them," said Hewitt. Some 35 percent of DSPs say that their work-life balance is worse or much worse than prepandemic, and 31 percent are working an additional 31 hours per week in overtime.

Hewitt highlighted recent legislation that could aid the workforce and offered some words of hope. The Build Back Better Act, for example, had important provisions regarding workforce development grants and technical assistance to states and providers. The American Rescue Plan Act also has provisions that offer states options for increasing compensation for DSPs and supporting workforce development strategies. She concluded her remarks by asking for programs that uplift and train the health care workforce to include DSPs in those efforts.

Discussion

Ayers opened by asking the panelists to talk about the cultural and systems issues they think need to be addressed before or while developing model workforce strengthening programs or competencies. Holder replied that it is imperative to address payment reform and reimbursements, encourage innovation in terms of greater efficiency with the available dollars, and break down silos as much as possible so that the workforce becomes more integrated. Havercamp seconded those ideas and added the need for real policy work to accelerate work at the local level and through grassroots efforts. She noted that the Institute for Exceptional Care is identifying policy levers that could improve training and health care quality.

In terms of cultural issues, Havercamp said it is important for health care providers to recognize that people with disabilities are vulnerable to social determinants of health and need culturally competent care. For Hewitt, the biggest need is to recognize DSPs, require training for them, provide salaries commensurate with their work, and create career pathways that allow them to stay in direct support roles but achieve greater levels of competence for which they would be paid more.

SPOTLIGHT PRESENTATION: OPERATION HOUSE CALL

In the first of three presentations about a promising program, Maura Sullivan (the Arc of Massachusetts) discussed Operation House Call, an initiative aimed at medical students to build confidence and interest in working with the IDD community and address the implicit biases that affect treatment and assessment. This program, said Sullivan, is reaching over 1,300 medical and graduate nursing students annually in Massachusetts and Connecticut with the help of over 250 volunteer families. These families, including hers, welcome students throughout the year into their homes for experiential learning opportunities. She noted that her two sons, who both have autism, grew up sitting on the laps of medical students from Boston University and Tufts University Schools of Medicine.

Every major medical school and some graduate nursing schools in Massachusetts and Yale School of Nursing in Connecticut participate in Operation House Call, which has four components. A parent instructor, such as Sullivan, gives a 2-hour, didactic lecture that includes an individual with IDD and their caregiver. The trainees also engage with panels of families, individuals with disabilities, and experts and make home visits, where the students spend a few hours with a family to experience what life is like with a disability and see what is ordinary and extraordinary for the individual and their family. In these visits, which transitioned to virtual during the pandemic, the students also learn what the individual's journey has been like in the health care community, what it is like for them to navigate in the community, and about their fight for equity and inclusion.

Finally, the students reflect on this experience in essays they post on an online, privacy-protected forum. "I spend a lot of time crying when I read these," said Sullivan, "because of the impact that these families and our course has made. [The students] see the strength in the individual, the resilience in the family, and they want to help. They want to learn more."

The program's learning objectives focus on communication and the importance of speaking directly to the person with IDD to build a bond and trust, even when they cannot respond. Other learning objectives focus on intersectionality, moving toward more culturally competent care, and monitoring bias and diagnostic overshadowing. Sullivan tells stories about her own sons, who have had incidents of aggression, self-injurious behavior, and sleeplessness, and how she wants health care professionals to look beyond those behaviors for the underlying causes. For example, one of her sons had severe gastrointestinal issues that, when treated, reduced much of his aggression and other challenging behaviors. Operation House Call also provides accommodations and tips from its 250 volunteer families.

The other aspect of Operation House Call is that it aims to get medical students to change the culture in which they work, both now and in the future. The goal is to have the medical students model the desired behavior by using language that puts the individual with IDD first, before their disability. As an example, she recounted an incident when her son Neil was having a challenging time in the ED and being aggressive and loud. When a parent told her to "put a muzzle on that thing," a doctor who heard that remark came over and said, "Neil, I am so sorry that you are hurting, and I am so sorry that you have to wait, but I am going to help you, and I'm going to help your parents, because you deserve it." He then looked around the room and made eye contact with people, and that changed everything. "Patients and staff were coming up and asking me how they could help Neil," said Sullivan.

She said she tells this story because she knows that medical students have the power to make that kind of impact but also because she wants them to think beyond a little boy like Neil to the adult with severe disabilities who might be in that same position, or an individual of color, or someone who does not speak English. "Can they step up and can they make that kind of change?" asked Sullivan, "because that is what we need."

While Operation House Call is a success in the short term, Sullivan said that health care professionals need this kind of exposure repeatedly through training they receive after medical school. She noted that the program is expanding to include training for ED clinicians. It will also have a final product to disseminate nationally by the end of 2021. The biggest challenge to the program has been sustainability, with most of its funding coming from donations and the Arc's fundraising activities and not from the medical schools. Another challenge has been that while medical students are enthusiastic and hungry for this experience, residents and practicing doctors are less so. However, given the increasing awareness about health equity and the issues that some medical providers have had complying with ADA requirements, Operation House Call is now getting requests from physicians who want this training.

CHALLENGES IN FINANCING AND PAYMENT

The day's third and final panel, moderated by Hoangmai Pham (Institute for Exceptional Care), discussed the challenges arising from financing—how money gets into the system—and payment—how money flows out to reimburse service providers. Pham noted that speakers in the previous panels had touched on the importance of financing and payment and how it can impede progress when done poorly. The three speakers on this panel were Michael Monson (Altarum Institute), Air Ne'eman (Harvard University), and Cheryl Powell (The MITRE Corporation).

Challenges in Financing Payment for People with IDD

Altarum, explained Monson, is a nonprofit organization focused on improving the health care of individuals with fewer financial resources and populations disenfranchised by the system, particularly older adults, women, children, military and veteran populations, and people with disabilities. Most of its work is with state and federal governments and focuses on turning policy into practice in four areas, all through the lens of health equity: transforming the service delivery sector, advancing public health, integrating public health and the service delivery sector, and scaling health infrastructure.

The key financing and payment barriers to enabling integrated, person-centered care for people with IDD are variations in the types of services covered, a lack of financial incentives for integrated care, and structural payment issues. Monson stressed that these are not the only barriers, merely the three major payment-oriented barriers. Other barriers include presumptions of fraud that exist in the system and limits on self-direction and how individuals can use funds.

The services that someone can receive depend on their insurance coverage. Medicaid beneficiaries, for example, have quite complete coverage across all the various types of services they might need, whether for physical health, long-term services and supports (LTSS), behavioral health, and pharmacy. Medicare beneficiaries only have good access to physical health services and pharmacy, with limited access to behavioral health services, which is also true for most individuals with commercial insurance. Individuals eligible for both Medicaid and Medicare—"dual eligibles"—get the best of both worlds, said Monson, and thus can access a fairly complete package of benefits.

Good coverage does not guarantee that a person will get integrated, person-centered care, because the incentives for providers to work together and provide such care do not exist in the fee-for-service system that dominates Medicare and Medicaid. For example, a state Medicaid program will make direct payments to a physical health or LTSS provider. "Each of those are getting separate payments, and neither have an incentive to work together or with other providers," which is particularly true when working together may result in lower payments and fewer services, even when the situation is better for the patient, said Monson.

Dual-eligible beneficiaries experience the same issue: the state Medicaid program will make direct payments to LTSS providers and behavioral health services, while Medicare pays the physical health provider and for pharmacy services. No entity, said Monson, works to coordinate care or provide a person-centered approach to assist the beneficiary.

However, financial alignment can create the conditions that can lead to more integrated, person-centered models of care: a risk-bearing entity, such as a managed care plan or a provider-led system, takes in Medicaid and/or Medicare payments and disperses the funds to the different provider types. In theory, that entity has the incentive to ensure more integrated, person-centered activity, because of the evidence that having greater access to HCBS and coordinating care reduce spending.

Legitimate concerns exist, said Monson, that risk-bearing entities might just hold onto the money and reduce services for people with IDD, which is why it is important to have strong governmental oversight for these types of models. The government's role is to ensure that these entities are, in fact, putting people at the center of care, that they are getting the services they need, and that they can appeal decisions that limit their access to services.

Monson noted that alignment of financial incentives via risk-bearing entities, by itself, may not facilitate person-centered care—especially if the payments to these entities is insufficient. Medicaid, for example, pays them on a population basis, which means they get the same payment for every individual in a similar population. This can lead to adverse selection issues (the population that the entity serves does not look like the average population). If a health plan has more people with IDD than average, it will not receive the funds to provide appropriate care for that population.

Medicare does something similar, but it pays risk-bearing entities based on each individual enrolled, using a "hierarchical condition category." These category scores are based on the beneficiary's medical record, and if the physician does not properly document all the health issues, the reimbursement rate will be insufficient. Moreover, this model does not fully account for the needs of people with disabilities and creates structural issues that systematically underpay risk-bearing entities for people with disabilities and those with IDD.

Finally, the way providers are paid does not adequately reimburse them for these populations, Monson emphasized. Physicians are reimbursed on a time-based system that is calculated on the average. Given the extra time physicians spend with people with IDD and other disabilities, the payment structure systematically underpays them. In addition, many physicians will not accept Medicaid beneficiaries because of the lower overall reimbursement rates that Medicaid provides versus other payers, and Medicaid is the predominant insurer for these populations. Taken together, these payment issues constrict the supply of providers that are available to care for individuals with disabilities, including those with IDD.

Monson identified clear opportunities to create more financial alignment and establish more appropriately governed risk-bearing entities and a need for Medicaid rate structures specific for people with IDD to deal with the adverse selection problem. Also needed, he said, are fixes in the hierarchical condition category risk adjustment model to properly account for the care of people with IDD; as noted earlier, if the physician does not properly document all of a patient's health issues, the reimbursement rate will be insufficient. Capturing appropriate data for people with IDD will help inform those rate structures and risk adjustment models. Enhancing payments to providers to reflect the time it takes to provider true, person-centered care for people with IDD is also required. The big challenge, he said, is that this payment reform will have to happen across the entire industry.

Measuring Quality in IDD Services

Reiterating Monson's point about the important role states have in exercising oversight on risk-bearing entities, Ne'eman said it is important to provide states and other policy makers with the proper tools to measure the quality of IDD services. He reviewed two models to thinking about disability. The medical model assumes that the problems of living with a disability are the inevitable result of biological impairment. For example, this model holds that someone in a wheelchair cannot enter a building because they cannot walk. The social model thinks about the challenges of living with a disability in terms of the interaction of biological impairment with a variety of societal factors, such as stigma, the availability of services, and public policies. According to the social model, that person only lacks a suitable ramp.

These are not just philosophical differences, said Ne'eman, because they determine how the system attributes causality and the responsibility for the problems and challenges people with IDD face during their lives. Ultimately, he added, these determine how to measure outcomes. "To know how providers and health plans are doing, we have to think about what is in the realm of possibility for them. What do we think they can realistically impact through service provision, through better case management, or any number of other things, and what problems do they simply inherit?" asked Ne'eman.

Looking through the medical model lens leads to policy solutions, such as risk adjustment of quality performance scores for providers, that hold providers and health plans harmless for taking on a more medically complex or more high-need population. While that is certainly an appropriate and necessary step, it will not close all gaps in outcomes; those gaps result from not only biology but systemic injustice. In that case, the social model emphasizes that plans should also be accountable for addressing the social disparities that people with disabilities face.

Until recently, said Ne'eman, relatively few National Quality Forum–endorsed quality measures focused on LTSS. Those that did often focused on institutional care, such as nursing homes, or behavioral health services in early childhood. The past 10 years, however, has seen HHS and disability stakeholders work to expand the number of quality measures for HCBS, creating opportunities to measure quality in managed LTSS through both survey instruments and measures that can be derived from administrative data.

This effort, he explained, builds on a long-standing literature on measuring quality of developmental disability services that focuses on surveys of people with disabilities and their families. For Ne'eman, the gold standard for this approach is the National Core Indicators Project, a collaboration of state agencies nationwide that not only asks questions regarding health and medical care but also speaks to key issues regarding autonomy, choice, control over one's own life, and whether people have their rights respected in various service settings.

Ne'eman cited a real fear on the part of self-advocates, families, and providers that managed care organizations may not have the proper expertise or may have financial incentives that do not lead them toward desired outcomes and values. Avoiding that requires quality measures that not only give some degree of accountability and transparency but can be tied in some way to financial incentives. In fact, many managed LTSS contracts now tie quality measure to financial incentives, including withholding portions of the capitated rate and requiring those organizations to meet quality measurement standards to receive those funds.

New York's financial alignment and dual-eligible demonstration for people with IDD had significant variation in the kinds of quality measures it emphasized. Some, particularly those in effect in the first year of the demonstration, focused on the plan, the ways it interacted with members, and whether the service plans documented member care goals. Other measures—particularly those in the later years—focused on outcomes, such as the proportion of people in state institutions who transitioned into the community or people with developmental disabilities who are directing their own services. These outcome-based measures, said Ne'eman, are where he would like to see the field focus in coming years, in part because they will speak to whether the shift from fee-for-service care is benefiting or creating more challenges for people with IDD. Toward that end, the Centers for Medicare & Medicaid Services (CMS) have introduced three sets of measures relating to rebalancing and use of LTSS that states could use for managed care contexts: assessing the rate of admission to an institution from the community, the proportion of admissions to institutions that result in successful discharges to the community, and the proportion of long-term institutional residents that transition to the community.

In summary, Ne'eman said that despite tremendous progress over the past 5 years, a number of areas still need more work on developing measures. "We still need to see more investment in measures that look at service experience, in particular the degree of choice and autonomy that people with developmental disabilities have and their ability to control the services that they receive," he noted. Also needed, he said, are measures for transitions within the HCBS spectrum, such as when people move out of group homes into supportive community living in their own homes or family homes as well as other, more integrated options.

The field is also at an early stage in measuring day services and employment service quality, said Ne'eman. He also pointed to the need for a broader conversation regarding when to apply a risk adjustment framework in terms of quality measures and when we want to apply it around closing disparities when thinking about disability.

The Swiss Cheese of Financing Services and Supports for People with IDD

Ideally, said Powell, financing should enable a care and financing system that supports individuals with IDD in attaining their goals by wrapping around their needs and preferences. The harsh reality is that even with the best health plan, the path is unclear, too many challenges prevent needed services and supports, and financing and payment mechanisms can be duplicative or nonexistent for some services and supports, all of which lead to suboptimal outcomes.

The holes in the financing system arise from two major factors, said Powell. One is that care services, financing, and payment are fragmented across multiple systems, which creates a lack of cohesion, shared vision, and agreement as to who should pay for what services. The second factor is that so much is unknown about how to best provide care, support, and services for people with IDD, let alone who should receive benefits. "Many people with IDD go unidentified to receive services because of data issues," explained Powell. "They may be identified in one program but not in another because of differences in data and differences in how the programs identify individuals with IDD."

In addition, it is still unclear what services are going to make the optimal difference in a person's life, how much to pay for those services, and how to measure success. Powell said that if the goal is for individuals with IDD to live their best lives, better measures are required that can determine if the services those individuals are receiving are helping them do just that.

Expounding more on the issue of fragmentation, Powell said that the IDD population's needs are served by disparate systems, including housing supports, workforce development, education, public health, health care, family and caregivers, transportation providers, and HCBS. In addition, different organizations and funding streams finance each of these systems, and these organizations often do not talk to one another or face obstacles that prevent aligning. This fragmentation leads to duplicated services, gaps in service, a lack of a shared understanding and vision, burdens for everyone, and unclear and suboptimal outcomes.

Some payers, such as Medicaid, are ahead in financing and paying for integrated IDD health care, supports, and services with partner organizations, but many payers are trailing behind or just getting started, said Powell. In her mind, financing and paying for holistic care for individuals with IDD is a team sport, and some of the rules need to be rethought or rewritten to enable the team members to work together. Medicaid and Medicare integration models represent one approach that seems promising, she said, as are the emerging ways in which funding streams are coming together across social services, education, and health care. She would like to see newly created payment methodologies that would incentivize partnership and service integration and other payers becoming interested in financing supports and services for individuals with IDD.

Powell listed a number of future strategies to fill the holes in the Swiss cheese financing system (see Table 1) but said that the best way to get to the ideal state she outlined is to bring together payers across the public and private sectors to work with the other sectors that deliver supports and services, creating streamlined financing that wraps around care management and care. The challenge is to have data that accurately identify individuals with IDD so that payers can finance the necessary services and incentivize how the different sectors provide them.

Discussion

Pham opened the discussion by asking the panelists about their level of optimism about adopting the appropriate financing and payment mechanisms in a health care system that is so profit driven. She noted that new data from the National Health Interview Survey indicate as many as 20 million people in the United States with IDD and wondered how to keep the growth of this

TABLE 1 Strategies to Address the Holes in Financing Services and Supports for Individuals with IDD

Current	Future
Few designated, public payers	Many payers across public and private sectors
Separate, disconnected funding streams	Thoughtfully integrated funding streams
Financing/payment and care management for social services and health care are often bifurcated	Financing/payment and care management for social services and health care are streamlined
Unable to identify people with IDD and finance/pay for services	Data accurately identifies people with IDD and is linked to financing and payment
Financing/payment support short term, program-specific goals	Financing/payment support vision of individuals with IDD living best lives
Payment methodologies and incentives are often disconnected from needs and goals	Payment methodologies and incentives drive toward care/service alignment with needs/goals
Payment disconnected from outcomes	Outcomes-based payment
Payment/services determined by providers/system	Payment/services determined by individual and caregivers

SOURCE: As presented by Cheryl Powell at the workshop on Optimizing Care Systems for People with Intellectual and Developmental Disabilities on December 10, 2021, Powell slide 7.

population from scaring payers either into passivity or ignoring them entirely because of worries about the cost of serving this growing population.

Monson replied that rather than being afraid of the profit motive, it should be possible to leverage it using the right quality infrastructure to measure if people with IDD are getting to live their best lives, to reward those plans that innovate and do things differently to achieve that goal. "I think we have to reframe the conversation," said Monson. "Profit is not necessarily a bad thing. Unregulated profit that we cannot measure outcomes against is a bad thing."

Ne'eman said he agreed that market incentives have a role, but he noted two important caveats. The first is that the current system is far from having plan financial incentives aligned with quality measures that address integration, choice, control, and autonomy, the things we care most about when it comes to HCBS. "Without good ways of measuring what we care about, we can't set financial incentives to promote those outcomes," Ne'eman argued. The second caveat is that most of the managed LTSS frameworks are not engaging in risk adjustments that adequately distinguish between types of disabilities or severity of impairment within particular disability categories. His concern is that without quality measures, managed care organizations will follow the path of least resistance and provide fewer services to stay under their total capitated payment rate or discourage higher-cost enrollees to make a bigger profit, as has occurred with some Medicare Advantage plans. Monson emphasized the false dichotomy that pits fee-for-service versus managed care. The challenge, he said, is creating the right system and using a quality measurement system for delivering IDD services.

In terms of how the disability community can keep government payers from running scared at the notion that this population is growing so rapidly and has such deep unmet needs, Powell suggested having the CMS Innovation Center assess whether this population will cause costs to skyrocket. She thinks this may not be the case, because these unmet needs may be driving higher health care expenditures. In that case, greater integration with other payers and social services and supports might lower costs. Moreover, getting people the care they actually need can reduce unnecessary costs and waste in the system. She feels that developing a more integrated system to provide care, support, and services for this population could identify ways of transforming the system for everyone and taking pressure off of the health care system.

CLOSING COMMENTS FOR DAY ONE

Some consistent contextual themes that several speakers noted, said Pham, included social equity, and what national initiatives exist to improve value in health care and how unsustainable the system is, and how timely it is to talk about these issues given the COVID-19 pandemic.

Another theme was the importance of paying attention to the stress on caregivers created by a system that makes families and caregivers feel isolated and responsible for solving all their challenges on their own. Too often, said Pham, they have to inject themselves into the system rather than having the system meet them where they are and take care of those needs. The core reason for that situation, she said, is a lack of respect for the basic humanity of individuals with IDD and an under-awareness and poor understanding of this population and what individuals with IDD need to live their best lives. The system should be responsible for helping these individuals get to where they want to be, and they should not have to fight so hard through the system to get there, said Pham.

Another theme Pham highlighted was the need to better prepare the workforce—clinicians and direct support providers—to serve the IDD population. Speakers emphasized the opportunity to professionalize the home- and community-based workforce and for organizations in that sector to work together, learn from one another, and engage in authentic partnership with individuals and their families. Pham identified a strong sense that exposure is what builds familiarity, eliminates bias, and opens up the possibilities for meaningful care relationships.

A fourth theme was that in the nation's push to move people with IDD out of institutions and into the community, it lost the expertise of health care professionals who had cared for them every day yet did not prepare the rest of the health care workforce or services and support systems to properly care for this population. As a result, the complexity of their needs and the reflex toward diagnostic overshadowing has ended up causing harm.

The speakers offered many different strategies for improving the clinical workforce, but those strategies will not be sustainable or scalable without fixing the financing and payment system and making hard policy choices that motivate service providers to get that training and give them a path that does not seem impossible to them, Pham summarized. The last panel covered the complexity of the financing and payment system and the bright spots that are addressing its shortcomings. Pham emphasized that it will be important to pay service providers fairly, in a way that leverages their profit motive constructively so that they are working toward goals that are important to people with IDD in their communities and accountable for achieving good outcomes. "Profit may be fine, but it has to be steered toward goals that are meaningful, acceptable, and of high value to the community," Pham said in closing.

DAY TWO: CURRENT AND PROMISING INTERVENTIONS

Pham offered some reflections of what she learned from the first day of presentations and discussions. The main lesson, she said, is that the system of care, services, and supports is far from optimal. It does not include all the services that people with IDD and their families need to live their best lives, nor is it easy for them to navigate. "What we are looking for is a system that is much more connected across the different service silos and that can do the work so that affected people and caregivers do not have to carry so much of the burden in navigating through that maze," said Pham.

Another lesson from Day One concerned the challenges associated with the clinical workforce and DSPs needed to provide HCBS. With that workforce, the challenge is to address the lack of cultural and technical preparedness to service this population, while the main issues confronting the workforce are severe stress, gross underpayment for the services they provide, minimal political support, and no clear path for professional development and advancement.

The final lesson of Day One concerned the challenge of providing adequate financing and payment for services that are based on actual need and not population averages. In short, the speakers acknowledged that the system needs to be tailored to individual needs and goals in a way that engages the affected community, hears their voices, and shares power with them in decision making. Beyond paying more for what individuals need, quality and outcome measures must be developed that can hold service providers in the system accountable for the outcomes that matter to individuals with IDD and their families. "Clearly, there is a lot of work to be done," said Pham, "but we also found the day inspiring because we heard about what is possible in terms of bringing more science and more political will and more resources to the problem."

INNOVATIVE MODELS OF CARE AND COORDINATION

Day Two began with descriptions of three illustrative models of care and service coordination. The three speakers were Clarissa Kripke (University of California, San Francisco, School of Medicine), Patricia Aguayo (University of Utah Health), and Lauren Easton (Commonwealth Care Alliance). Elizabeth Mahar (the Arc) moderated an open discussion.

The CART Team

Kripke and her colleagues in her institution's Office of Developmental Primary Care developed the CART team as a multidisciplinary mobile consult service focused on serving adolescents and adults with IDD, their clinicians, family members, and support professionals (Kripke et al., 2011). The idea behind the team, which disbanded when its funding ended, was to fix system issues while identifying the population's complex medical and services needs. The team included experts in developmental primary care, nursing, psychiatry, psychology, and caregiver support with a combined 100 years of experience supporting successful community living, and it served clients from six northern California regional centers. Services included phone and e-mail consultations, clinical assessment and consultation, training and technical assistance, advocacy, and online resources.

As an example of the CART team's clients, Kripke recounted consulting about an autistic young adult who was constantly violent and responsible for a great deal of property destruction. When the team observed him in his home, it realized that his "attacks" were involuntary, a tic that was stereotyped and predictable. The team's main intervention was reinterpreting his behavior in neurological rather than behavioral terms and moving him to a larger home with fewer roommates. The team also arranged for him to transfer to day services focused on interesting activities rather than trying to get him to inhibit movements beyond his control.

In another example, a client was expelled from school because of self-injurious behaviors and a lack of progress. The school was implementing what it thought was an evidence-based intervention for nonspeaking autistic individuals with a system of picture icons. However, this young woman was blind and deaf, and English was not spoken in her home. The intervention was to connect the family with regional experts in tactile sign language and address cultural issues, such as her mother feeling uncomfortable with male home health providers when her husband was at work.

One client the team saw could not access medical care because he would be agitated and aggressive, shattering windows in a car and attacking clinic staff. The team communicated with him directly, something that his service providers did not think was possible, and learned about his trauma as an immigrant, being separated from his family, and history of moving from unsuccessful home to unsuccessful home. In his experience, getting into a car usually meant that he was going to abruptly lose his home or be subjected to restraint or painful medical procedures.

The CART team program, said Kripke, was successful in helping people with complex needs, but it shut down because it could not secure permanent funding once its start-up funding ended; it could not predict when referrals or patients would come in, so it could not sustain a dedicated team. The disability agencies Kripke and her team had contracted with during the pilot phase were not willing to risk offering sustainable funding in a contract because they feared it was not eligible for HCBS funding. She noted that such funding is supposed to respond to the needs of individuals, which the program did, but the team's goal was to be proactive rather than responsive and to serve the population instead of only individuals by working across silos to improve the environment in which people were seeking care. "It is very hard to stabilize people if we wait for them to be traumatized repeatedly," she explained.

One of the most common issues the CART team addressed was dealing with medical professionals who underestimated the prognosis and quality of life for people with disabilities, which frequently led to attempts to premature withdrawal of lifesaving care, said Kripke. She noted that the team remained focused on practical problem solving, drawing on the large body of training materials she and her colleagues have developed. These materials include forms to track seizures and medication administration along with toolkits on communicating with individuals with IDD and supported decision making, and disability-sensitive sexuality training.[11] The team also engaged a client's primary care providers and caregivers in problem-solving activities, without making recommendations that the clinicians or caregivers could not implement, and provided ongoing support to overcome barriers to implementing any recommendations.

Kripke explained that the team's medical recommendations sometimes included diagnoses, pills, and procedures but often involved changing a person's environment or LTSS. "Generally, we were well received by clients, families, and medical professionals, and we were valued by the service systems who felt supported to resolve complex cases without institutionalization," she said.

Kripke offered that while the CART team story might sound like a good argument for Medicaid managed care organizations to take on long-term care service contracts as a way to better integrate medical care with long-term care services and supports, that is not the answer. "If there is an entity that assumes risk, it should be government entities or nonprofit organizations focused on disability services and run for and by people with disabilities," she said. As an example, she cited California's Regional Centers System, for which the state assumes the risk, and some model disability care organizations.

The problem is twofold, said Kripke. First, involving Medicaid managed care organizations quickly becomes a race to the bottom to provide the worst possible care for the most complex and expensive patients. As soon as it becomes expensive and complicated, she explained, these organizations will try to get patients to go somewhere else. Both profit and nonprofit managed care organizations figure correctly that absorbing a loss on a patient or a small subpopulation is less expensive and easier than actually solving their complex problems.

The second problem with using Medicaid managed care organizations to fund long-term care is that it undermines 50 years of disability advocacy

---

[11] Available at https://odpc.ucsf.edu (accessed April 29, 2022).

work, said Kripke. Managed care organizations that focus on acute medical care are fundamentally geared toward providing medically necessary services chosen by health care professionals. Long-term care is not about diagnosing and treating illness but rather about providing services and supports aimed at maximizing potential and participation. People with disabilities and those who support them, not health care professionals, choose those services and providers, she said, who might be family members rather than professionals. Disability services and supports are different missions and require different skill sets and operations than health care and are rooted in different paradigms and value systems than managed care organizations. "A managed care organization focused on medically necessary care is not concerned about how many days of work you miss because you have been stuck in bed without a wheelchair repair or whether you had transportation and an aide to attend a holiday meal with family," said Kripke. "They only care if you end up in the hospital with a pressure sore, because if you don't, there are no cost savings."

When she started this work, Kripke thought managed care organizations would be interested in improving health service delivery for people with developmental disabilities because it is a high-cost, high-risk population. Now, after 20 years, she knows that changing quality measures or payment structures is not a powerful enough incentive to get such an organization to fundamentally change its primary mission, which is driven by the medical model of disability. "Changing something so fundamental to their business, their values, and their mission to provide medically necessary care recommended by doctors is a heavy lift, and it only benefits a handful of their members," she said. She noted that expenditures for people with IDD are a small part of the overall expenditures of a general Medicaid population.

Kripke cautioned that despite the potential value in integrating acute medical care with long-term care for better coordination, maintaining mostly separate systems that can hold each other accountable is also valuable. "We spent the last 50 years separating the disability services system from the health care system for a good reason," she said. "When health care providers and systems have total control over everything a person with a disability needs to survive, history tells us that that really does not end well. People grounded in the disability community recognize that as regressive policy being couched in progressive language."

Healthy Option, Medical Excellence: The Huntsman Mental Health Institute Neurobehavior HOME Program

The Healthy Options, Medical Excellence (HOME) program was created in 2000 as a partnership between the University of Utah Departments of Psychiatry and Pediatrics and with funding from the Robert Wood Johnson

Foundation and an agreement with the Utah Department of Health. "We were trying to show how, when given the right opportunity, we could provide for these high-spending populations," Aguayo explained. Since then, the program has demonstrated that it can cut costs, and Utah has renewed its agreement every year.

The HOME program serves as a colocated medical home that provides medical and mental health care to children and adults with IDD. It operates as a Medicaid managed care organization funded through a fee-for-service arrangement, explained Aguayo. The program bills internal services through its Epic electronic health record. The university health plan processes the billing and credits the program statistically.

Philosophically, the HOME program aligns as closely as possible to the principles of the patient-centered medical home model to provide comprehensive, patient-centered, coordinated, accessible, quality care. Eligible individuals must be Utah Medicaid beneficiaries, have a documented IDD and mental health or behavioral concern, and be willing to receive primary care at the HOME clinic. As of November 2021, 1,367 people were enrolled. Aguayo noted that the program treats the most behaviorally and psychiatrically complicated patients in the community.

Aguayo said the "secret sauce" of the program is its care management. Each enrollee has a case manager as the point person and problem solver for all concerns, whether medical, behavioral, or school related. The case manager, she explained, has immediate access to the entire team and is able to rally necessary supports and services and respond with a solution within a few hours. When a crisis arises or things are challenging at home, case managers help support the parents, with whom they become quite close. In addition, case managers are in charge of bringing into the care team those in the community that the team feels are important, such as teachers or schools.

The program encourages all enrollees, even those who are stable, to come to the clinic at least every 6 months, get a physical exam once per year, and meet with a psychiatrist at least once a year, even if they are not taking psychotropic medications. Every morning, the entire clinical team meets to discuss patients who may be struggling, so that everyone is aware of the situation, and those who are hospitalized for medical or psychiatric reasons.

The other component that Aguayo said makes the HOME program unique and successful is that it is a lifetime partner, providing pediatrics, family medicine, and geriatric services. "We serve patients throughout their life, and that allows us to have seamless transitions," she said. The program does its transitions slowly, she added. "We start talking to patients in pediatrics about transition around 16 or 17, and not just about the transitions within the clinic but throughout all of these things that are involved in their life," said Aguayo. The transition process includes bringing in agencies or community partners who may be involved in those transitions, be it guardianship, group homes, schools, or job support agencies. Even the team's psychiatrists, who are child and adolescent psychiatrists, stay with the individual throughout their transition to adulthood. Recently, though, the HOME project hired a geriatric psychiatrist; the transition to them starts between age 45 and 50, and they will follow the patient and manage their medications until the end of life.

The HOME program offers a wide range of in-clinic services, including primary and psychiatric care; individual, group, and educational therapy; occupational therapy and behavior analysis; psychological testing; and dietary services. For any external services or referrals to specialists, the program tries to stay within the University of Utah health system to allow for easy collaboration and communication and take advantage of a common electronic health record. Aguayo noted that the program has strict formal documentation and quality measures so that it can show the state how it is doing, what services it is billing for, and how it is growing its services. It is only serving the Salt Lake metropolitan area, though it does have some members in rural or remote parts of the state who come to the clinic once a year. During the pandemic, telehealth enabled the program to improve delivery of some of its services to rural communities.

The program has been successful at keeping its clients out of the hospital by providing them with excellent medical and psychiatric care. In fact, the probability that a HOME enrollee will require hospitalization drops as their time in the program increases. Psychiatric and medical readmissions within 30 days of initial discharge have also decreased over time. "We try to keep that low by collaborating closely with an inpatient team and ensuring we have a good transition back to the community," said Aguayo.

The biggest strength of the HOME program, she said, is the way it collaborates with families and caregivers and acts on the feedback it gets from them. For example, parents have liked the newly introduced virtual model of care introduced during the COVID-19 pandemic, and the program will continue that in some form, though it will still ask clients to come into the clinic at least once a year. "We want patients to be familiar with the setting and with their providers so that they are comfortable," said Aguayo. "Once they have been here a couple of times, they are comfortable in that environment and they participate in their care consistently."

Flexibility in terms of care adapted to each individual's needs is a program strength. For example, the team will meet the client in their car or allow a break during an appointment if that makes them more comfortable. Strong partnerships with community organizations is another strength, as is the seamless transitions as a client ages. Continuity in care and quality improvement activities are important program attributes, as is the staff's expertise in IDD. Aguayo said she could not stress enough how important the program's relationship with the state and legislature has been. "They are the ones that have maintained this program going and are part of our partners to make this continue as a program," she said. She added that an external agency runs the monitoring and audit program.

Regarding challenges, Aguayo pointed to the program being restricted to Medicaid patients and its limited geographic catchment area, both of which are dictated by the state, the shortage of qualified professionals, and adequate triage of the clients the program serves.

Optimizing Care Systems for People with IDD

Commonwealth Care Alliance (CCA) opened in 2004 as an integrated care system for individuals who were eligible for both Medicaid and Medicare benefits, said Easton. It is both a payer and provider that has over 40,000 members across Massachusetts who represent the state's population with the most complex care needs. Over 70 percent of its Senior Care Options members are nursing home certifiable yet able to live safely and independently at home with the program's care and support. Over 65 percent have four or more chronic conditions, 60 percent have a physical and/or behavioral health disability, nearly 60 percent primarily speak a language other than English, 53 percent have diabetes, and over 9 percent have a major physical disability, such as paralysis, spinal cord injury, multiple sclerosis, muscular dystrophy, cerebral palsy, or ventilator dependency (CCA, 2021).

For CCA's One Care Program, which serves dual eligibles aged 21–64, 76, ~70, and ~32 percent have a major physical and or behavioral disability, mental illness, or a substance use disorder, respectively. Nearly 9 percent have a major physical disability such as paralysis, spinal cord injury, multiple sclerosis, muscular dystrophy, cerebral palsy, or ventilator dependency, and over 7 percent are homeless or marginally housed. The cost of caring for the One Care–eligible population averages seven times the average cost for MassHealth's managed care organization patients.

What makes CCA different, said Easton, is that every individual drives their own care plan and has a dedicated care partner. CCA does an annual face-to-face assessment for the care plan. Every member also has access to the full complement of an interprofessional care team comprising licensed and supportive clinicians and a health outreach worker who functions like a community health worker. The teams coordinate their activities across the continuum of care and support individuals who may be in residential homes or living at home and their caretakers. CCA also works closely with the Department of Developmental Services and the Department of Mental Health to provide coordination and collaborative partnerships with community providers. Central to all of this is a recognition of the member's autonomy, dignity, and voice.

Program engagement, explained Easton, focuses on developing comprehensive, longitudinal relationships between individuals and their care partners to establish trust with individuals who may not have had the best experiences with the health care system. CCA's integrated model includes primary, medical, palliative, and behavioral health care, addresses social determinants, provides LTSS and acute episode management, and manages prescriptions. CCA emphasizes a community-focused, de-medicalized care plan that integrates environmental and community supports, shifts the site of service to the community, and promotes independence. This comprehensive approach has decreased health care utilization and produced better outcomes, with reduced care gaps, stabilized behavioral health issues, improved polypharmacy and medication adherence, and decreased ED visits, hospitalizations, and readmissions.

CCA has developed several innovative programs for its complex client population. For the approximately 5 percent of its members who do not have a primary care clinician, it created the Wrap Care model that stratifies members into structures most appropriate for their needs and pairs each patient with a One Care partner based on individual medical, behavioral, and social needs. CCA's full-spectrum primary care program offers support for high-risk members that goes beyond what a traditional practice provides. This program focuses on members who do not thrive in a traditional primary care model because of their physical and psychosocial disabilities. In addition, a mobile interprofessional team of on-demand, multidisciplinary clinicians augments CCA's care partners through direct care delivery, coordination, and consultation. This team provides episodic support and on-call services after hours.

The InstED program uses specially trained paramedics to respond to and triage a member's urgent care needs in their own homes, avoiding unnecessary ED visits. The paramedics communicate with on-call staff and evaluate and treat members in their own residence. For members who require hospitalization, CCA's Hospital to Home program provides medical expertise and care coordination across care settings while enhancing patient experience (CCA, 2019). Located at the inpatient setting, this program provides medical consultation with insight on individual members and expertise on caring for members with complex medical and psychosocial needs, particularly those with disabilities.

The Life Choices Palliative Care program serves as an alternative to traditional hospice by providing a broader range of in-home services throughout the course of serious illness, not just at the end of life. CCA's palliative care registered nurses work closely with care partners.

One program that Easton started is the Crisis Stabilization Units, two unlocked crisis units (totaling 26 beds) that help members in an acute behavioral crisis stabilize and avoid hospitalization. A full-time licensed clinical social worker and psychiatric nurse practitioner staff the units, which offer rehabilitative and recovery-focused services.

CCA will open an engagement center in the first quarter of 2022 that will provide a community-based, trauma-informed alternative to ED settings for members with subacute needs. The center will identify and assist members with overwhelming social determinants of health that result in psychiatric and/or medical admission and create an environment of meaningful intergenerational interaction that will decrease isolation. The center's goals will be to address gaps in required assessments and facilitate peer leadership and development. The hope is to provide members with the opportunity to come to the center and get help from staff and peers to deal with social determinants, behavioral health needs, and substance use needs. The center will have recovery coaches and behavioral health clinicians on site.

Discussion

When Mahar asked the panelists if any of them changed their models based on community feedback, Kripke said that her program has been influenced heavily by its partners, coworkers, people with disabilities, and its clients. In fact, self-advocates wrote many of its training materials. She explained that her program partners with self-advocacy organizations that are integrated into all its activities and its interactions with patients. Aguayo reiterated her earlier remark that her program has incorporated more telehealth services based on feedback from patients and parents, adding that this option has reduced no-shows. Easton's program has Member Voices, a group of members that inform and drive CCA's clinical models. This group was involved from the outset in developing and implementing the new engagement center, and it helps decide what technology would help with the clinical model.

Given the panel's diverse experiences with and views of risk-bearing organizations and providers, Mahar asked them about potential value in offering a range of different arrangements from which members can choose. Easton replied that CCA has incorporated what it calls "help homes," human service providers and community health centers that CCA provides with a per-member, per-month payment so they will perform care management. These providers and health centers have existing relationships with some clients that CCA does not want to disrupt. Aguayo said that her program does not offer much choice. Kripke said she believes that people with disabilities should always have access to whatever is available to the general population, and if they do enter a program that is specific to people with disabilities, that should be voluntary.

Mahar asked the panelists about opportunities and barriers to scale their models. Aguayo said that her program depends on the state to scale its program and that the state dictates its catchment area. That said, her team is working on how to provide services to rural areas, perhaps by establishing satellite clinics. Kripke said that primary care has to be local but also identified a need for regional services, perhaps linked via telehealth or through mobile clinics, for those areas where expertise in care of people with developmental disabilities is scarce or nonexistent. Easton added that her program faced some challenges in scaling as it grew from 1,000 to 40,000 members over the last 7 years. She also noted that CCA is an expensive, though incredibly effective, model because of its use of advanced practice clinicians who go into patients' homes.

Responding to a question about how CCA finances its activities, Easton said that it benefited from Massachusetts being one of the first states to enact a dual-eligible program, so it receives funding through Medicaid and Medicare. Each individual receives an assessment, which drives CCA's rating and risk categories and determines its per-patient, per-month payment.

An audience member asked the panelists if they see the COVID-19 pandemic as an opportunity to advocate with CDC to declare people with IDD as a medically underserved population. Kripke responded that they are a medically underserved population, but getting that designation involves a political process that was reviewed recently and may not be revisited anytime soon. Aguayo suggested that partnering with state government could be key in making that change possible, an idea Easton seconded, given that her program is working with state officials to expand access to the One Care program.

Mahar asked the panel members about other elements that they would like to include in their models. Aguayo replied that there are too many to count, but one feature she would like to add is the crisis units that Easton described. Easton said she would like to add housing with integrated support and care, an idea Kripke supported.

SPOTLIGHT PRESENTATION: BUILDING A BEHAVIORAL THERAPY METAVERSE

Ravindran (Floreo) explained that his company is leveraging the power of virtual reality to provide a method of teaching social, behavioral, communication, and life skills for individuals with autism spectrum disorder and related diagnoses (Parish-Morris et al., 2018; Turnacioglu et al., 2019). This approach adds virtual reality to telehealth to provide richer experiences that go beyond videoconferencing.

After playing a short video showing how virtual reality therapy works, Ravindran explained that the company works with 100 providers who use this tool. The company is also innovating on new pathways to allow families to use it. Floreo has accomplished this through Medicaid waiver programs in Maryland, Wisconsin, New York, and Washington, DC, that take advantage of assistive technology reimbursement to adopt new technology that can benefit their patients. This supplement enables parents to receive the full system and provide therapies on their own schedule without the logistical challenges of getting their children to the clinic.

The company's goal, however, is to create more scalable reimbursement channels, said Ravindran (Ning et al., 2019). The ideal situation would be to receive regulatory approval so that providers could prescribe this system as a type of therapy, which might lead to a seamless process for reimbursement through health plans. Another possibility is for CMS to authorize bundled payments for behavioral health supports so that families can self-direct resources. A third path would be to allow broad coverage and payment for telehealth services and enact cross-state licensing reforms that would allow businesses to build telehealth options that they could offer more broadly. Ultimately, Ravindran noted, this can only happen if every family has access to broadband.

Given that virtual reality is emerging as a new therapy medium, for not only autism but areas such as pain relief and anxiety, it will be important to recognize it as a form of therapy that merits its own coverage policies and Healthcare Common Procedure Coding System codes. In addition, payers will have to accept that the infrastructure costs that providers might take on to offer it will pay off in terms of better outcomes for the families they serve.

INNOVATIONS IN WORKFORCE SOLUTIONS: THE ROLE OF GENERAL HEALTH CARE PROVIDERS

As an introduction to a session on innovative workforce solutions to meet the needs of individuals with IDD, Susan Thompson Hingle (Southern Illinois University School of Medicine) said she hoped the three panelists would discuss efforts that could lead to a more equitable world in which those with IDD, such as her son, would receive optimized treatment. The panelists were Kristin Sohl (University of Missouri and ECHO Autism Communities), Lisa Howley (Association of American Medical Colleges), and Sarah Ailey (Rush University College of Nursing). Following the presentations, Hingle moderated a brief discussion session.

ECHO Autism Communities

Many individuals with IDD, autism, and other types of disabilities are, in general, served in academic medical centers, said Sohl, which means having to go to an urban center that offers better access to best practices or specialists. In addition, it is often higher-income families who are able to access best practices and specialists because they can take time off from their jobs or travel. These factors lead to increased health disparities for many individuals based on socioeconomic status, racial and ethnic identities, geographic location, and gender. Sohl also noted that while specialty centers are phenomenal places that can serve many individuals with IDD, that does not mean they serve everyone.

Generalists, she explained, do not get much formal training about IDD, which means that a pediatrician or family physician may feel ill equipped to properly treat an individual with IDD or support the family. The challenge then is to establish systems of care to improve the health and well-being of individuals with IDD and other types of disability that go beyond specialty clinics in urban centers. The model she and her collaborators developed, ECHO Autism, is based on the Extension for Community Healthcare Outcomes (ECHO) model[12] developed at the University of New Mexico that at its core is about moving knowledge, not people. Her team began adapting this model to apply it to autism and other disabilities in 2014.

The ECHO model addresses the challenge practicing physicians face in recognizing when they have to start learning something new or need additional support and guidance. ECHO does this by using technology to amplify and leverage scarce resources, sharing best practices to reduce disparity, adopting case-based learning to master complexity, and using a Web-based database to monitor learning outcomes.

Sohl's program focuses on using the ECHO model to leverage the scarce expertise available for individuals with autism and their families. It starts with physicians/practitioners presenting their real cases to an expert hub team that helps them learn. She stressed that the heart of this model is the relationship that develops between expert mentors and generalist learners and how that can benefit patients. For example, as a specialist in autism, she has a great deal of knowledge about evaluation, diagnosis, and longitudinal care for someone with autism and other developmental disabilities, but she does not know the individual patient or their community. When done right, the interaction between teachers and learners creates what Sohl called a "learning loop," where the expert team learns from the local care teams while providing ongoing mentorship and guided practice for the generalists, who can then work more effectively and feel more competent to treat individuals in their communities.

Sohl stressed that this is not telemedicine. ECHO Autism is different because 30–40 primary care clinicians from around the country might join one of the twice-monthly, 90-minute sessions to learn about primary care in

---

[12] Available at https://hsc.unm.edu/echo/what-we-do/about-the-echo-model.html (accessed April 28, 2022).

the autism space. The focus is on teaching primary care clinicians to identify individuals with autism spectrum disorder and to screen for and manage common medical and psychiatric problems. The primary care clinicians, in turn, take that new knowledge and apply it in the populations they are serving. The goal is to accelerate the process of disseminating scientific discoveries into best practices that all clinicians can use. This approach, she said, democratizes expertise and disseminates best practices to mentor and guide communities of clinicians, educators, and advocates, creating local expertise and increasing access to optimal care for individuals with autism and their families. ECHO Autism is also active in the advocacy and policy arenas to hardwire changes into the system to deal with reimbursement and access issues.

Sohl and her collaborators have been building ECHO Autism communities across Missouri, and today, all children in the state live within 45 miles of an ECHO Autism primary care clinician. "That means families are not traveling around the state to try to figure out where they can go to get answers," said Sohl. "They can get answers right in their home community." Now, she and her collaborators are expanding their ECHO Autism programs to provide professional development and guided practice to colleagues in psychology, early intervention, mental health counseling, crisis intervention, caregiver skills training and family/self-advocacy. Regarding the latter, the idea is to help a local/regional support group leader, for example, learn how to better support their community using the same case-based learning approach.

As of June 30, 2021, ECHO Autism had 170 communities in Missouri, 88 communities spread across 30 states and the District of Columbia, and communities in 10 countries. It has teams of experts or specialty clinicians at some 50 U.S. institutions and 20 international locations, all of which coordinate their activities through her group at the University of Missouri. In the year ending June 30, 2021, Missouri-based ECHO Autism programs had 667 participants, including 514 from Missouri and 153 from outside of the state. "What I hope this shows you is that peer-to-peer mentoring or expert-to-generalist partnerships—guided practice, if you will—is powerful and can start to move knowledge and reduce stigma related to the care and service of individuals with disabilities and autism," said Sohl.

Her team is also developing resources for generalist practitioners, educators, and mental health professionals so that they can access best practices quickly and easily. Sohl noted that every ECHO Autism program is open to anyone who wants to learn about best practices for caring and serving individuals with autism and other IDDs.

Medical Student Education

The Association of American Medical Colleges (AAMC), said Howley, is a member of a new diverse action collaborative called "ABC3,"[13] or Action to Build Clinical Confidence and Culture by the Institute for Exceptional Care, which will scale strategies nationally to engage and better prepare general clinicians for serving people with IDD. For AAMC, this means transforming medical education to improve care for those with IDD. To effect change in a medical school curriculum, it is important to understand how accredited medical schools are governed and how decisions about curricula are made. Howley shared some brief background information into how medical education works, given the frequent misconceptions within and outside of health care.

Medical schools that offer an M.D. are accredited by the Liaison Committee on Medical Education (LCME), which is jointly sponsored by the AAMC and the American Medical Association (AMA) and recognized by the U.S. Department of Education as the organization responsible for accrediting medical schools. There remains a strong firewall between the accrediting body and the functions of the member organizations, the AAMC and the AMA. The goals of the accreditation process are to protect educational quality and encourage its improvement, Howley explained. LCME provides standards and guidelines to medical schools for their educational programs, but it does not mandate specific practices or have a standardized set of practices within or across these programs. There are 12 accreditation standards, each with an accompanying set of elements.

For example, one standard requires every medical school to have a group of individuals who oversee a program as a whole, including the curriculum. This curriculum committee is ultimately responsible for the educational program at an institution's educational sites, and it oversees what is taught and how the curriculum is structured. Diverse educators, learners, patients, and community partners have an important and increasing role on these committees and supporting the work that they do in overseeing competencies, competency development, learning effectives, curriculum implementation, assessment, and evaluation, said Howley.

She discussed two additional standards: faculty of a medical school must define the competencies or outcomes that students should achieve, and faculty must ensure that the content is broad and deep to prepare their learners for entry into any residency program and their subsequent contemporary practice of medicine. In addition, Standard 7.6 states that the medical curriculum includes content regarding the "recognition of the impact of disparities in

---

[13] Available at https://www.ie-care.org/abc3 (accessed May 16, 2022).

health care on all populations and potential methods to eliminate health care disparities."

In recent years, medical education has been shifting to a competency-based approach for teaching and learning. Over the past two decades, medical education has improved in the way it defines outcomes, such as competencies, and how it uses them to guide teaching and learning, said Howley. Competency-based education, which has its roots in primary education and psychology, is a way of thinking about designing and facilitating education; despite no single model, common characteristics include a relentless focus on outcomes and a shared language. She reminded participants that Havercamp presented the core competencies on disability for health care education during the first day (ADHCE, 2019). "We are delighted that these competencies are now available to help inform broadly our medical education community, and I strongly encourage you to refer to them and use them as you're developing and enhancing curricula," Howley stated.

She noted, too, that AAMC will soon be issuing a new set of relevant competencies on diversity, equity, and inclusion that it expects will serve the full continuum of medical education, including faculty already in practice and those instructing the students and residents in training. These competencies focus on the broader issues and include expectations that physicians will advocate for inclusive and equitable practices and physical environments, anti-ableism, mitigating other biases and health communication, and many other actions. They are designed to encourage collaborative discussions on diversity, equity, and inclusion and disabilities.

Howley offered that AAMC has two journals, *Academic Medicine* and *MedEdPORTAL*; the latter publishes stand-alone, complete teaching or learning modules that have been implemented and evaluated with medical or dental trainees or practitioners. AAMC has also published a report, *Accessibility, Inclusion, and Action in Medical Education, Lived Experiences of Learners and Physicians with Disabilities*, that provides guidance on how to improve the learning climate within medical schools for students with disabilities (Meeks and Jain, 2018).

Howley also offered three takeaways:

- Medical (and health professions) education is a complex and continuously improving process.
- Competency-based education is an optimal approach to teaching and assessing physicians across the continuum from medical school to practice.
- Input is needed on how to better design, share, and research better models to ultimately improve care for all patients, including those with IDD.

Partnering to Transform Health Outcomes for Persons with IDD

Partnering to Transform Health Outcomes with Persons with IDD is a workforce development program funded by a 5-year grant from the Administration for Community Living under provisions of the Developmental Disabilities Assistance and Bill of Rights Act (DD Act) and led by a national consortium of organizations, explained Ailey. The program's goal is to integrate high-impact learning and practice materials, developed in collaboration with the National Center on Interprofessional Education, into interprofessional education programs at the five core partner institutions starting in the third year of the grant. The plan is to disseminate those materials to an additional 35 institutions in the fourth and fifth years.

Underlying this effort is the need for social change, said Ailey. "Persons with intellectual and developmental disabilities face systemic discrimination and dehumanization in the health care system," she said. "Look at what happened at the beginning of COVID-19, when most hospitals immediately jumped to denying persons with disabilities the right to have a support person with them when hospitalized." Her institution was an exception, instituting a policy in early April 2020 that anyone who needed a support person could have one. The Office of Civil Rights issued a statement in June making clear that persons with disabilities had a right to a support person in the hospital.

In talking to some people, Ailey said a common thought was that denying loved ones' access to the hospital was a good thing. "My reaction was, this is reprehensible," she said. "You are actually making things worse, but there is all too often a disconnect between how health care professionals view themselves as being in caring professions and then what they actually do. To me, to get change, we have to create a sense of outrage."

Ailey said the project's collaborators are using the Collective Impact Model to organize their work and the spirit and provisions of the DD Act and the phrase "nothing about us without us" as guiding principles. Groups wanting to achieve social change use the Collective Impact Model, which brings together multiple stakeholders, including those directly affected, to drive social change by working together on a common agenda (Ennis and Tofa, 2020). This model recognizes the potential power differential among stakeholders and has strategies to assist putting everyone on the same footing. Beyond a common agenda, four other conditions of collective impact exist: shared measurement, mutually reinforcing activities, continuous communication, and backbone support (Ennis and Tofa, 2020). Ailey noted that in keeping with its "nothing about us without us" philosophy, the program established an advocacy advisory committee to enhance the participation of advocates in the steering committee and action networks, provide another avenue for input, and support one another.

In the program's first year, Ailey and her collaborators organized a steering committee and three consortium action networks focused on communication; education, practice, and policy; and measurement, evaluation, and outcomes. The three networks include about 50 active participants, including advocates, health care professionals from multiple professions, health care professional educators, people specifically involved in interprofessional education, representatives of organizations involved in relevant policy and services related to persons with IDD, and policy makers.

The communication action network has created a website. A content strategist was hired to develop multimodal messages, said Ailey. The education, practice, and policy action network leads the program's work to develop and acquire high-impact materials on addressing community–academic interprofessional education partnerships. The measurement, evaluation, and outcomes action network has been leading an environmental scan and literature review on the state of practice in education health care professionals and identifying materials to go into toolkits for posting on the program's website for dissemination.

One reason the program is focusing on interprofessional education is that it is impossible to achieve change at the necessary scale by educating one profession at a time. In addition, a paradigm shift is occurring in health care that is moving health care professional education toward interprofessional education. In part, this paradigm change is connected to the growing recognition of the need to address the social determinants of health. Another reason for stressing interprofessional education is that in the real world, teams deliver health care, which works best if the members of the team bring their own discipline-specific knowledge and skills while acting as members of the team. That dual identity, said Ailey, is the main concept of interprofessional education.

Health care professional education is delivered mostly in silos of the different professions, with students of several professions (e.g., medicine and nursing) receiving their training in specific hospital units and on specific services. "This system of education does not meet the needs of persons with intellectual and developmental disabilities, nor, for that matter, the needs of health care systems in the 21st century," said Ailey. "We need health care professionals who address improving health, working with persons with intellectual and developmental disabilities, their supports, and health care workforce in the community, such as direct support professionals, and we need health care professionals capable of providing episodic, acute care in complex conditions of care."

Ailey said that the program's five core institutions are developing community–academic partnerships to create planned situations so that students can experience and address health inequities as part of their training. The program is also training community health mentors, community members with IDD who will participate in telehealth visits with the interprofessional student teams. At her institution, all students across all disciplines complete a two-trimester interprofessional education program based largely on the geriatric interdisciplinary team training initiative (Fulmer et al., 2004).[14] Her institution is now working with persons with IDD to craft stories about what is important to them and their health; it includes them as part of program's training and posts them to its website.

Program evaluation, said Ailey, will examine both individual- and community-level outcomes, determined in partnership with the community. The program will identify the components of interprofessional education that can become longitudinal projects for student involvement across their education.

Developing longitudinal projects will be based, in part, on experiences at Rush. For example, in 2007, her institution established an interprofessional committee tasked with improving hospital care of persons with IDD. Over the past 14 years, some 100 students from medicine, nursing, occupational therapy, speech therapy, and health systems management have worked on related projects. Ailey discussed capstone and other projects at Rush designed to address issues in care that the students must complete to graduate. Ailey noted that while the projects are short and usually focused on one issue, they have collectively influenced her institution's culture and the long-term community-based projects. She added that the Agency for Healthcare Research and Quality has a documentary on Rush programs posted on its website.[15]

Her hope is that the program will build disability-friendly health systems in the same way that the geriatric interdisciplinary team training initiative, which The John A. Hartford Foundation has funded since 1995, has created geriatric-friendly health systems.

Discussion

Hingle asked the panelists to identify some of the policy levers and actions that accrediting bodies could take that would help scale their programs. Sohl said one needed reimbursement policy change would allow primary care practitioners to spend the necessary time to meaningfully care for people with IDD. The other factor that affects scalability is the stigma associated with IDD

---

[14] Additional information is available at https://www.johnahartford.org/grants-strategy/geriatric-interdisciplinary-team-training-program-resource-center-nyu (accessed April 28, 2022).

[15] Available at https://www.healthmattersprogram.org/2020/05/13/none-of-us-want-to-stand-still-documentary (accessed April 28, 2022).

and the lack of awareness and understanding, something that training can address. What she has found in her work is that as soon as someone starts to better understand IDD, they become open to taking care of more individuals with disabilities.

Ailey replied that working with multiple stakeholders can help with scaling these programs. As an example, she cited the work that multiple governmental, community-based organizations, advocates, and health care professionals did approximately 8 years ago to develop a health resume that is now part of the Epic[3] electronic health record and available nationwide. This same coalition also partnered with the organization that developed the Health Risk Screening Tool (a web-based rating instrument to detect health destabilization in individuals with IDD) to integrate it into an Illinois version of the Health Risk Screening tool, which means it will be mandatory for every group home in Illinois to use it.

From an educational perspective, Howley said that a consensus is developing around the competencies that trainees should gain in diversity, equity, and inclusion. These competencies could be used collaboratively to guide curricular development or review existing activities that include training on improved communication, reduced bias and stigma, and other person-centered clinical skills for those patients with IDD.

Hingle asked the panelists to discuss cultural training opportunities that would address bias toward individuals with IDD. "How can we start to train people to make the experience of interacting with patients who are from the IDD community more joyful?" asked Hingle. Ailey replied that this is not an easy task, and she recalled being at a presentation at which the presenter put up a headline concerning someone with a disability who had some awful experience. "If this headline said the person was Asian or African American or gay, there would have been outrage at what happened," said Ailey, "and there is not any sense of outrage when you talk about what goes on with intellectual disabilities."

Sohl agreed with Ailey and said that changing culture takes leadership to set an example of how everyone and everyone's abilities matter. When she thinks back on her medical education and how her perspectives on disabilities have changed, she knows that it was because she had good people whom she could learn from and model. Sohl said this comes back to the "nothing about us without us" philosophy and seeing people for what they can offer. One problem with the medical model is that it focuses on what people cannot do, an attitude that perpetuates stigma. "The more we can embrace what can be done, what can that person contribute, what can they say for themselves or do for themselves, the more we can really lean into and lead a new generation that accepts people for exactly what they bring to the table," said Sohl.[16]

INNOVATIONS IN FINANCING AND PAYMENT

The final session of the second day featured three speakers who addressed innovative financing and payment models and the quality measures needed for those models to succeed. The speakers were Brede Eschliman (Aurerra Health), Sarah Hudson Scholle (National Committee on Quality Assurance [NCQA]), and Stephanie Rasmussen (Sunflower Health Plan). Hoangmai Pham (Institute for Exceptional Care) moderated a discussion after the three presentations.

Innovations in Payment and Financing for IDD Services

Aurerra Health Group, a mission-driven health policy and strategic communications consulting firm with nationally recognized experts in alternative payment model design and implementation, was tasked by the Institute for Exceptional Care to develop a series of case studies on innovative payment and financing mechanisms for people with IDD. The goal, said Eschliman, was to learn about the current state of innovation, highlight promising models, and identify any missing elements.

Financing, explained Eschliman, is where the money comes from—a budget or appropriation of a total amount of money available to compensate providers. Common health care financing mechanisms include the Medicare trust fund and premiums, copays, and employer-sponsored health insurance. Payment is the compensation made to a person or entity for a service (how a provider is paid). Fee-for-service, a typical form of payment in the United States, involves a provider submitting a claim and an insurance company reimbursing them.

Innovation pertaining to financing and payment involves paying for services in a different way, paying for different services, or restructuring financing or payment across silos in a way that improves quality of care and quality of life, said Eschliman. An example of paying for services in a different way would be to move away from a fee-for-service model to an accountable care organization model in which Medicare assigns a population of patients to a group of providers and gives them a benchmark payment equal to the expected costs of those patients for the year; if costs are under that benchmark, they

---

[16] Information available at https://www2.illinois.gov/sites/icdd/Investments/Pages/Better-Communication-Better-Health-Care-Campaign.aspx (accessed June 15, 2022).

share the savings with the accountable care organizations or that group of providers. The provider group bears the risk of keeping costs at or below the benchmark payment.

As an example of paying for different services, Eschliman cited the Got Transitions pilot program that paid providers for a transition meeting between a pediatric provider and adult provider who would be taking over the care for an adolescent or young adult. Most health plans do not cover this service. She also noted the Massachusetts General Hospital Down syndrome program, which convinced an insurance company to cover an app that helps primary care providers who do not have expertise in Down syndrome understand the screenings they should perform and services they should provide for their patients with Down syndrome.

To illustrate a model that restructured financing or payment across silos, she mentioned an autism clinic that receives its funding from a commercial health plan and uses some of that funding to support staff so they can attend individualized education plan meetings between families and schools. In this case, funding meant for health care is also supporting a nonclinical school service. "That is a small example, but when you think about this population, there is a wide range of services that typically have different funding streams, and an example of innovation would be figuring out a way for those to work together a little bit better," explained Eschliman.

Turning to the three case studies she wanted to present, Eschliman started with the Lee Specialty Clinic, which provides multispecialty care that includes primary care, as well as dental, podiatry, ophthalmology, physical therapy, nutrition, audiology, crisis intervention, and other services to patients with IDD ages 13 and up in Louisville, Kentucky. Insurance claim payments only cover about 25 percent of the cost of running this clinic, which Holder discussed in his presentation on Day One, with the rest of the funding coming from the state. The Kentucky state legislature annually appropriates a budget for the clinic, which passes any claims reimbursements on to the state.

This is a unique financing mechanism, said Eschliman, because states do not typically allocate money to cover the types of health services outside of Medicaid that this clinic delivers for its clients with IDD. It is also unique in that funding is divorced from individual claims, which guarantees that the clinic will have enough money for all of its services regardless of claims to insurance providers.

The second case study she discussed was the Utah Neurobehavior Home program, a clinic in Salt Lake City that provides medical, psychiatric, and chronic care management services to children and adults with both an IDD and a mental health or behavioral health diagnosis. The University of Utah functions as both a payer and provider. It runs a Medicaid managed care plan that receives a capitated payment from the state, and providers in its network are employed by the university. The university can use the lump sum payment to provide health care services without having to wait on payment for individual claims, though it does submit what Eschliman called "pseudo-claims" to its own insurance plans for tracking purposes rather than payment. In addition, this program is a financing innovation in that it consolidates separate Medicaid funding streams for physical health services and mental or behavioral health services. It convinced the state to provide a single payment to cover all of those services so that it could deliver its care model in a more holistic and less fragmented manner.

The Penn Autism Clinic was the third case study. This model is unique because the clinic functions as part of the employer-sponsored health insurance plan for University of Pennsylvania employees. The clinic conducts intake and assessment for children and young adults who have or are suspected to have autism spectrum disorder and are covered by the employer-sponsored plan. It develops care plans for other providers, tracks progress on those plans quarterly, and helps families with individualized education program meetings with schools. This is a function that insurance companies often refer to as "utilization management," and it is unique to have an independent clinic perform it. Eschliman explained that this is a payment innovation because the health plan covers the full cost of the clinic through its internal budget. It is not a financing innovation, because typical mechanisms, such as premiums and copays, finance the health plan.

In preparing these case studies and conducting interviews with eight other organizations with interesting programs, Eschliman and her collaborators identified some common themes. The first was the opportunity for true creativity in this space, given the few alternative payment models and appetite for new, creative ideas. It is promising that the providers and payers they interviewed have not been forced to wedge IDD services into alternative payment models designed for other populations but instead think creatively about what they need for this specific population. A second promising theme was the large amount of drive and willpower in this space, often from people who have personal connections to IDD and are willing to put in an incredible amount of time and effort into being creative about payment and financing models.

The third promising theme was that payment models tended to put the care model first and then design the money around it. She commented that when she worked for the Center for Medicare & Medicaid Innovation (CMMI), it would develop alternative payment models and financial incentives and hope that the perfect care model that improved quality of care would flow from these.

The early evidence showing that these innovative models reduce hospital costs was the final theme Eschliman noted. Interviewees emphasized that people with IDD are often underserved, which means that a goal of paying for different types of care would be more appropriate than a goal of lowering the total cost of care. Many of these programs, though, had early evidence of their payment model reducing hospital costs, which she said is a great sign.

What is still missing, she said, is scalability beyond the committed core of people who work in the IDD space. The success of these models, said Eschliman, is often limited to what those people, through sheer force of will, are able to implement on their own. Unless they have champions, the models are not scaled. Another limitation is that these innovative plans do not cover HCBS. Those that do tend to involve restructuring the state agencies that administer programs more than doing innovative things with payment.

The lack of comprehensive data within or across the organizations that provide services for people with IDD is another missing element, as is the limited variety of innovative models that organizations have developed and tested. The case studies she discussed were variations on cost-based reimbursement, and many programs require a special waiver from the government or legislation. Having a greater variety of models would allow researchers such as her to test the effectiveness of models against one another. This might attract payers who have not yet been interested and, in particular, could allow for more experimentation with tying payment amounts to quality outcomes, which is not something that she has seen with many of these models.

Person-Driven Outcomes

The organization that Scholle works for, NCQA, creates quality measures that payment and financing systems use to determine whether models are achieving the goals for their individuals along with policy goals. She said that NCQA has been working for almost a decade to determine how best to measure quality for people with complex needs in places where traditional kinds of quality measures do not work, particularly for determining whether a health care system is helping people do what matters most for them in their lives. This effort initially focused on older adults and people with functional disabilities, but NCQA has seen a great deal of interest and enthusiasm around applying this approach with the IDD population.

As she understands the problem, the current system provides fragmented care and non-standardized and competing accountability structures, all of which make it hard to determine whether the investments different systems are making are paying off. This fragmentation will continue to get worse as states move to integrate people with IDD into managed care and the aging population grows, said Scholle.

NCQA thinks about measuring the quality of LTSS and whether a care system is serving its population well in terms of structure, process, and outcomes (see Figure 9). NCQA has structure-related products and uses them to accredit health plans and community-based organizations that provide LTSS case management. Some of these accredited organizations serve people with IDD. Measures that assess process look at whether an organization is conducting a comprehensive assessment and developing a comprehensive care plan.

For Scholle, the most exciting measures are those that evaluate whether the health care system is helping individuals achieve what is most important to them. She explained that NCQA defines a person-driven outcome as an outcome that an individual, or their caregiver if the individual cannot do it on their own, says is important to them. "Our thinking about this is that this outcome should be something that is identified in the care process and used for care planning," said Scholle. "It is something the individual is driving and it is helping promote their own engagement in their health and well-being." Person-driven outcomes measures, she added, integrate clinical care and measurement.

NCQA has structured ways of documenting this goal of care, by using either a person-reported outcome, such as a structured tool that assesses

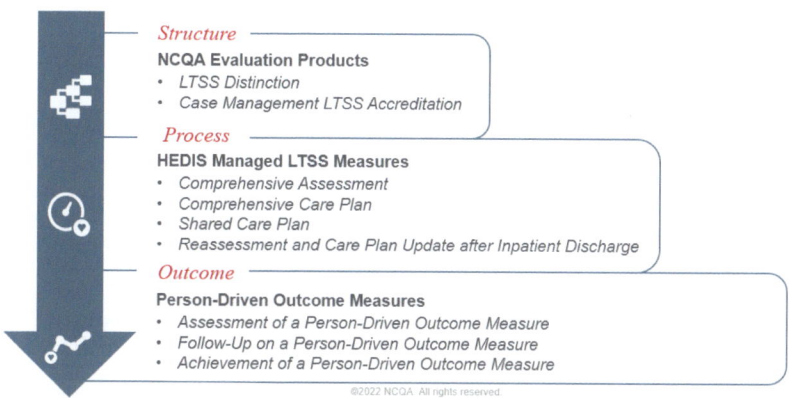

FIGURE 9 NCQA's LTSS quality framework.
NOTE: LTSS: long-term services and supports.
SOURCE: As presented by Sarah Scholle at the workshop on Optimizing Care Systems for People with Intellectual and Developmental Disabilities on December 10, 2021; Scholle slide 3.

physical functioning or somebody's engagement with care, or "goal attainment scaling," a structured approach where the individual and their provider jointly choose a goal and document and track it using a continuum of five possible outcomes: *much less than expected, less than expected, expected, better than expected,* and *much better than expected.* The care team uses this goal to develop action steps and then assess and adjust them so that those actions help people achieve what matters most to them.

NCQA has proposed three person-driven outcome measures (see Table 2). One looks at whether a health system has assessed and documented a person-centered outcome in a structured manner. Another examines whether the health system has followed up on that outcome after a specified interval of time to track and monitor the outcome and improve service delivery if needed. The third measure looks at whether the health system has achieved the person-driven outcome based on the personalized approach.

Scholle said NCQA has used this approach with over a thousand individuals at over a dozen settings. The focus has been on case management programs that span health and LTSS needs, including Medicaid case management for individuals with functional disabilities and for serious illness programs. Results so far show that these measures are working; they are seeing variability across sites. "We have rave reviews from individuals and care teams who have participated, and we have had everyone from a peer navigator to a physician involved in helping to document these outcomes," said Scholle. Most exciting

TABLE 2 NCQA's Proposed Person-Driven Outcome Measures

	Numerator	Denominator
Assessment of a Person-Driven Outcome	Documented person-driven outcome, using goal attainment scaling or person-reported outcome measure, AND a documented plan for achieving their individualized outcome	Individuals with an identified complex care need
Follow-up on a Person-Driven Outcome	Documented follow-up on the person-driven outcome within 180 days from the start of the measurement period	Individuals with an identified complex care need who had a documented person-driven outcome
Achievement of a Person-Driven Outcome	Documented achievement of the person-driven outcome (which can be maintaining or improving) within 180 days from the start of the measurement period	Individuals with an identified complex care need who had a documented person-driven outcome and follow-up

SOURCE: As presented by Sarah Scholle at the workshop on Optimizing Care Systems for People with Intellectual and Developmental Disabilities on December 10, 2021.

of all, she added, is that people exposed to this approach to documenting outcomes may be less likely to have expensive hospital stays and ED visits. None of these programs, she offered, specifically address people with IDD, but feedback suggests that this approach could work for this population. She also noted that NCQA is working to implement these measures in a digital environment.

Innovative Value-Based Contracting and Alternative Payment Models

To begin the final presentation, Stephanie Rasmussen said that Sunflower Health Plan, located in Kansas, is owned and operated by Centene Corporation, which has government health plans in all 50 states covering 25 million individuals. Centene's purpose, she said, is to transform the health of the community one person at a time by focusing on whole health, not just physical health, and forming partnerships in local communities that bridge social, ethnic, and economic gaps. The company has health plans in 13 states that manage different types of LTSS for about 346,000 individuals, with some 13,600 beneficiaries in Kansas, including those in seven online, community-based waiver programs and nursing facilities. Centene also manages IDD supports for individuals across 14 states, covering all benefits under health plans in Iowa, Arkansas, and Kansas. In Kansas, Sunflower Health Plan covers 53 percent of individuals with IDD who receive HCBS and 80 percent of those in intermediate care facilities for individuals with IDD.

Sunflower Health Plan currently has several value-based contracts and alternative payment contracts for providing care and services to its IDD population. She noted that Kansas has four primary providers who specialize in providing services for individuals with high-risk, challenging behaviors and medical needs. Her organization met with those providers, who said that part of their challenge was that they had to reapply for the state's higher reimbursement rate for residential and day services for individuals that have high-risk challenging behavior or high-risk medical needs. This made it hard to maintain the staff (clinicians and direct caregivers) and specialized programs needed to successfully support these individuals so they could remain in the community. To solve this problem, her organization created an alternative payment contract that essentially lends the funds they would receive from the state, which has enabled them to continue to provide services to these individuals and take additional referrals from her health plan for individuals at risk of being placed in a state hospital or private intermediate care facility. This contract, said Rasmussen, has been in place since 2016 and proven to be effective at ensuring ongoing access to that level of support for individuals who otherwise might be institutionalized.

Her organization also has value-based contracts for transition coordination services for individuals with IDD who are moving out of nursing facilities or private intermediate care facilities. Payments are based in part on readmission rates within the first 30 days of discharge. Rasmussen's health plan also has value-based contracts with several IDD service providers based on moving individuals with IDD from day services to competitive employment. The providers receive incentive payments 30 days after an individual becomes employed, when the individual remains employed after the first 6 months, and after the first year if the individual remains employed.

Currently, her organization is talking to its provider network about adding future outcomes to their value-based contracts, such as whether a job meets an individual's lifestyle preferences and if they are on the career path they want to follow. Other areas where discussions are occurring with IDD providers around value-based contracting include reducing gaps in care, expanding coordination of care using project ECHO approaches, reducing inpatient stays and institutionalization, workforce enhancements, and quality-of-life measurements.

Discussion

When asked how her organization is addressing the workforce shortage problem, Rasmussen said that she has been working with providers to access Federal Medical Assistance Percentage funding to provide retention and recruitment bonuses. A longer-term approach might be to expand the use of technology with individuals with IDD, to both decrease the number of staff that it takes to implement high-quality care and increase their level of independence.

Another approach is to look at high-quality service models that require fewer caregivers, such as when an individual with IDD chooses—and she stressed that this must be a deliberate choice—to live with or near their caregiver, who receives a salary or contract for holistic care. This usually results in higher-quality care, because fewer people are involved, and fosters stronger relationships when done well. "We are looking at developing a best practice manual and toolbox for how that service could be expanded in the state of Kansas," said Rasmussen.

When asked why her organization focused on employment as an outcome of interest, Rasmussen said that first, offering employment to young adults who are transitioning out of school who want a job is the right thing to do. Second, the data show that individuals with IDD who have jobs have better health and quality-of-life outcomes. Also, employment gives them a sense of accomplishment and self-purpose, which helps their mental health, and it reduces their reliance on more traditional IDD day services, reducing costs.

Pham asked the panelists to comment on the entities that they believe should be accountable when thinking about financing and payment. Eschliman replied that in the interviews her team conducted for the case studies, most of the responses laid that responsibility at the feet of health care providers. While she did not have an answer for what would be the best option universally, every organization interviewed said the accountable entity should be one that individuals and their families trust to have their best interests at heart and that develops care models that work for them and help them meet their goals. Pham wondered if, when an individual provider is the entity a person trusts to support navigating services, financing and payment should flow through that provider. Eschliman said that some models work that way. Wisconsin, for example, has multiple options, some of which include self-directed dollars. Her one caution was to be careful about predatory behavior and getting patients to declare that a certain entity should receive payments.

Scholle responded to Pham's question by stating that accountability is the flip side of responsibility. "What you hope to do through your payment models and quality measures is have the true north be something that makes sense to the individual and where the different providers or organizations that are involved in someone's care are all working toward that same true north," she said. That, she added, is what accountability models do when they work; ultimately, if things go well, the accountable entity is the responsible entity. She also noted that the hard part for people with IDD, as it is for people with complex needs, is that the entity trying to bring all the different providers necessary might not have the ability to get everyone going in the same direction. An individual clinician probably has little opportunity to be the service coordinator, while a health plan does but might not be as close to the person as a provider is. Pham summarized that idea as the care model has to come first, with financing and payment following.

Pham asked the panelists to discuss what is missing in terms of payers other than Medicaid participating in payment and financing of care for individuals with IDD. Scholle said the problem is that it is difficult to identify people with IDD from typical health care data, something that is true for all disabilities because of the different ways health care datasets capture disability status. Scholle wondered if some attributes are unique for people with IDD or shared with other complex populations that could help researchers such as herself define individuals with IDD as a subgroup.

CLOSING COMMENTS FOR DAY TWO

Perrin concluded the second day with his highlights, starting with the promising and different multidisciplinary models of providing the coordinated care that can help those with IDD and other complex health conditions lead their best lives, as well as some of the funding challenges they faced. Another highlight was the discussion of new ventures in health professional education, particularly those that engage groups of health care professionals to work and learn from each other through care experiences. Curriculum development was another topic he found interesting, particularly regarding competency-based education that optimizes care for people with IDD and reduces the stigma associated with IDD.

Perrin thought the discussions on payment and financing raised some of the challenges to creating models that incentivize high-quality health care for individuals with IDD and developing the measures for accountability. He noted the work on developing measures of person-driven outcomes and whether health care is delivering the things that matter most to individuals, as well as some imaginative strategies for developing value-based contracting.

DAY THREE: LOOKING FORWARD

The final day focused on where to go next. Perrin noted that the workshop planning committee had asked the day's speakers, when preparing their presentations, to envision what a blue-sky, brighter future would be for the IDD community.

CONSIDERING A NEW VISION FOR MODELS OF CARE

For the day's first panel, the three speakers imagined what care models could look like for people with IDD to help them get to a better place of health and health care justice and equity. The three panelists were John Kitzhaber (Foundation for Medical Excellence), Sharon Lewis (Health Management Associates), and Charlene Wong (Duke University). Kara Ayers and Alicia Theresa Francesca Bazzano served as co-moderators for the discussion session following the three presentations.

Elements of System Transformation

Kitzhaber believes four elements are essential for creating new visions for a model of care: giving oneself permission to imagine, being clear about the end goal, avoiding putting people into categories, and not underestimating either the importance of the community or the difficulty in building true community engagement and empowerment. Regarding the first element, the question he asks is, "If anything was possible and we were not constrained by funding, by partisan politics, or by the existing framework of statutes and regulations in which we operate, how would we create an optimal system for individuals with intellectual and developmental disabilities?" He noted that it can be difficult to answer because it can be hard to break free from a programmatic and organizational and institutional mindset, both of which limit creativity and imagination.

For example, all the major steps in health system transformation that Oregon has achieved over the past few decades, including creating the Oregon Health Plan and the state's Coordinated Care Organization model, required federal waivers for implementation because Oregon was not trying to achieve incremental change within the constraints of a deeply flawed system. "We were asking instead, if we were to start over, would we actually design a system that looks like the one we have today? The answer is obviously no," said Kitzhaber.

Being clear about the end goal means being clear about the problem being solved, he said. "Are we talking about an optimal health care system, or are we talking about a system focused on optimizing health, because they are not the same thing," he explained. For decades, said Kitzhaber, the national health care debate has defined the issue very narrowly as a coverage problem, so the question policy makers have been asking is how to achieve universal coverage. He considers that the wrong question, and as Thomas Pynchon wrote (1973, p. 251), "If they can get you asking the wrong questions, they don't have to worry about the answers."

Framing the problem narrowly as a coverage problem also narrows the solution space. To Kitzhaber, the right question is how to ensure that all Americans have a fair and just opportunity to be as healthy as possible, with health being a state of complete physical, mental, and emotional well-being, and not merely the absence of disease and infirmity (WHO, 2020, p. 1). He also called into question the veracity of the statement that health care is a basic human right, which assumes that health care is synonymous with health and that health runs exclusively through the health care system, both of which are untrue. "While access to acute care medicine is important, medical care itself is a relatively minor contributor to lifetime health status, and we have known that for decades," he said. Far more important, he added, are the social and economic determinants of health.

The policy implications of reframing the statement "health care is a basic human right" to "having a fair and just opportunity to be as healthy as possible is a basic human right" is to recognize two things. First, everyone has to have access to some level of effective, affordable medical care to be as healthy as possible. Everyone also needs the opportunity to achieve their full potential in a much broader sense: to have access to good housing and nutrition, safe communities and nurturing relationships, and education and meaningful employment opportunities, Kitzhaber explained.

His observation is that it will be difficult to build a system that optimizes health for individuals with IDD, or anyone else for that matter, by continuing to categorize people into separate groups, which contributes to bias and stigma. The federal Medicaid program, he noted, is mind-numbingly complex, with 28 mandatory and 21 optional eligibility categories that create an expensive and complex administrative nightmare, but it pigeonholes people into groups. "It seems to me that people should not be viewed and treated differently because of some arbitrary category," said Kitzhaber. "On the contrary, we need to view them as individual human beings, and our system must meet them where they are and address their unique issues and challenges." Only by doing that, he said, will everyone have a fair and just opportunity to be as healthy as possible and meet their full potential.

Kitzhaber then showed two pictures that have hung on his wall for 25 years and continue to be a source of inspiration. The first shows a young girl with IDD that he met during his first term as governor, and the second shows her on the day she graduated from a public high school. "She did not graduate from high school because she was in a category," he said. "She graduated because she wanted to graduate, because she was determined, and because she had the support of her family and her friends and a school that was committed to the success of each and every one of its students."

As Kitzhaber noted, the factors that have the greatest effect on lifetime health status and on quality of life occur outside the medical system. They take place in the family, in the home, and in the community. This means that addressing the social determinants of health, which he said are also the primary determinants of opportunity, requires a fundamentally different community-based delivery system and workforce. In his view, achieving both is the greatest challenge to creating a true health system as opposed to a clinically focused medical system.

While a community might have different agencies, programs, and community-based organizations and institutions providing services and supports that in one way or another seek to address the social determinants of health, these diverse entities are often dealing with only one major determinant at a time. Programs are often fragmented and operating in silos, with few if any coordinated handoffs between programs and services. In addition, the entities often have to compete for the same funding streams. Turf issues abound, said Kitzhaber, and organizational survival often takes precedence over the larger purpose for which these organizations and programs exist.

"We all pay lip service to care coordination, and yet true coordination requires dozens of programs and organizations and institutions and agencies and the people that work in them to be willing to subordinate their institutional, organizational, and programmatic interest to serve a larger common purpose," he said. That common purpose is the long-term success of the individuals these organizations serve, and serving that purpose requires putting those individuals in the center of the equation and ensuring that they do have a fair and just opportunity to be as healthy as possible. It also requires two difficult changes: transferring ownership and decision-making authority to the community and empowering those who are most impacted to play the central role in shaping the nature of the programs and the services and the investments they need.

Moreover, serving that purpose requires that members of the community must trust the frontline workforce and that people who make up that workforce must have a great knowledge of the community. Satisfying those two requirements allows these workers to serve as liaisons between the community and the medical system and social services. "This workforce is critical because it provides the connective tissue that makes possible a true, community-based health system, one that can indeed optimize both health and the opportunity to thrive, which in my experience go hand-in-hand," said Kitzhaber.

He offered that while it is impossible to change the direction of the wind, it is possible to adjust the sails and reach the desired destination. "I believe that destination is a society in which everyone has a fair and just opportunity to be healthy and to be all that we can be," said Kitzhaber, "and it seems to me that our responsibility here is to help all those in this country who face barriers and obstacles, whatever those barriers and obstacles may be, to adjust their sails—and ours—and to catch the wind and arrive in that port safe and triumphant."

Rethinking Holistic Coordination, Connections, and Integration for People with IDD

The work that Lewis addressed involved seeking a new vision for care coordination for people with IDD, including conducting an environmental scan and literature review, stakeholder interviews, and examining U.S. and international models with the goal of building a blue-sky vision of coordination that goes beyond the medical system or Medicaid HCBS.

As she and her colleagues looked at care coordination and case management, they found few formal taxonomies that look holistically at how to ensure coordination focuses on both the health system support needs that an individual has and community-related elements, valued social rules, and opportunities to achieve health. "For people with IDD, these are things that do not always evolve naturally and have to be supported," said Lewis. One of her favorite taxonomies was developed by New Zealand for individuals with brain injury. It notes that it is critical to not only meet people's health-related supports and services but help them reach their goals related to participating in life roles.

For this project, Lewis and her collaborators moved away from the idea of case management and terminology, such as "care coordination," centered around medical care. She noted that some stakeholders said that they negatively associate the word "care" with medical models, a deficit-based orientation, and paternalism because "care" tends to focus on solving a medical issue rather than helping someone achieve the life they desire. She pointed out that people with IDD are a heterogeneous population with a wide range of needs across the life-span.

Little surveillance and prevalence data broadly capture where people with IDD receive their services, said Lewis. Most are likely participating in publicly funded health coverage, but in some states, as many as one-third of the individuals with IDD have commercial insurance.

The New Zealand model uses local area coordinators, which it describes

---

BOX 1
A Working List of Holistic Coordinated Functions

- Information and referral
  - Helping people learn about, and find their way to, services and supports
- Eligibility and enrollment
  - Helping people understand and meet requirements to access certain programs or services
- Assessment
  - Listening, gathering information, identifying needs, and helping people share what is important for them
- Person-centered planning
  - Working with people to discover what is both important to them and for them, and trying to match supports and resources to their needs, interests, preferences, and goals
- Support plan documentation
  - Creating, updating, and keeping track of formal plans for support based on assessments, person-centered planning, and system rules
- Individual engagement
  - Actively listening to the person, offering comfort or empathy, helping them solve problems, supporting self-determination, self-efficacy skills development, and increased confidence
- Circles of support
  - Helping to develop and engage other people important to the person (family, friends, community)

as "walking alongside people with disabilities and their families to help people live good everyday lives within welcoming communities." It integrates financing and resources from multiple sources to support health, social services, community participation, and engagement for all people with disabilities in an area. Notably, she said, the model relies on not a single intervention but a set of interdependent actions that are designed, communicated, and delivered in an organized way intended to achieve the person's goal, address their preferences, meet their needs, and improve how they see quality of life.

Lewis's team defined a list of best practice functions that they compiled from multiple frameworks, stakeholder interviews, and various models, such as those discussed at this workshop (see Box 1). When they categorized those

- Coordinating and communicating
  - Working with the person, their family/friends, providers and others (representing systems or domains – health care, education, social services, employment, housing, technology, etc.) to make sure all of the pieces fit together (cohesion)
- Systems navigation
  - Actively helping people find their path through systems, paperwork, complicated processes to access goods, services, or supports, or to get their needs met in other ways (including assistance with self-direction)
- Monitoring health and safety
  - Making sure that people at risk have the support and help they need
- Service oversight
  - Making sure that people's services and supports are doing things according to their interests, needs, plans, and goals and the rules of the system
- Advocacy
  - Serving as an ally and an advocate when a person asks for help to make their voice heard, fix a problem, protect their rights, or address other needs
- Decision support
  - Helping people get and understand information they need to make their own informed choices, and helping them communicate their decisions
- Transition assistance
  - Anticipating changes whenever possible, and making sure that when change is happening, supports are adapting as needed

SOURCE: As presented by Sharon Lewis at the workshop on Optimizing Care Systems for People with Intellectual and Developmental Disabilities on December 14, 2021.

functions, they fell into four sets of actions: assessing and planning, engaging and facilitating, collaborating and coordinating, and monitoring and documenting.

One issue that came up repeatedly in the literature review and stakeholder interviews, said Lewis, was a concern about the competing goals and interests when health insurance and managed care entities take on risk to provide these functions and inherent tension with utilization management and delivering supports in a person-centered manner. "When we start thinking about some of the monitoring, documenting, quality measurement, utilization, and efficiency efforts, those are important but they need to sit separate and apart from the coordination effort," said Lewis. "Coordination should represent and support the person."

Lewis commented that when she and her collaborators interviewed stakeholders, they asked what characteristics and skill sets would make for a great coordinator. Nearly every stakeholder said that a great coordinators would be accountable to the individual and family and walk alongside them. One interviewee, Lewis said, described a great coordinator like a great orchestra conductor who helps the individual and the musicians in their life to play their chosen music in harmony. She then reminded the workshop that when talking about the long term with respect to people with IDD, that means birth to death, not the next 7–10 years. In that regard, part of what people are looking for is someone to be the historian, to have that longitudinal relationship and be on the life path with them.

The stakeholders also raised their need for adequate information technology and communication infrastructure so that the teams working on coordination and supporting the individual can share information timely and effectively. Lewis said that people get tired of telling their stories over and over again. They also made the point of keeping gatekeeper functions separate from the advocacy, coordination, and support person who walks alongside them.

Lewis agreed with Kitzhaber's comment about the need to rethink the types of organizations that have to be involved, how they fit together, and how they have to be willing to be more collaborative and less concerned with their turf and resources. Importantly, she said, funding needs to come from multiple sources, and the health system needs to be a partner, supporter, and engaged team member but not the driver of the coordination function. "Our advice to purchasers and to medical providers would be to help the broader community find ways to support people to have a holistic and cohesive approach to health and not base it primarily in clinical care," said Lewis in closing.

North Carolina's Integrated Care for Kids Model

For Wong, an integrated model of supporting health includes three intertwined components: holistically understanding the needs of a person and their family; providing support and bridge services that wrap around the person and their family, rather than asking people to wrap around systems; and focused and innovative health care investments on what matters most for individuals with IDD and their families. The first component, said Wong, requires health care data that exist mostly within silos, as well as data from sectors outside of health care. North Carolina, for example, is using data that individuals and their families are providing about prioritized social drivers of health, including food, housing, transportation, and interpersonal violence. She noted that the state asks these questions universally of all Medicaid beneficiaries and is working with some of the large private payers to bring them onboard. Her team is even looking at how they could have schools and early care and education centers ask similar questions of their families, and the state is building a platform that might eventually support universal screening for social determinants of health using data integrated from multiple sectors.

In addition to universal screening, a blue-sky model would make it as easy as possible for any individual, including those with IDD, to enroll in programs for which they are eligible, which is not always the case today. "By integrating cross-sector data, we can find opportunities to match individuals who are eligible but not enrolled and then cross-enroll them in programs," said Wong. North Carolina, for example, is looking at data from its Women, Infant, and Children program and its Medicaid data to identify people who match into multiple programs for which they are eligible but not enrolled and that are important for their overall health and well-being. She added it is important to use an equity lens when thinking about holistically understanding a person's and family's needs. Unfortunately, she said, data are often not disaggregated by equity variables, including race, ethnicity, disability status, or language preference. As a result, part of thinking about a blue-sky model requires considering how to facilitate collecting those data as a critical first step to developing evidence-based policies and effectively implementing disability-inclusive policies and programs.

As examples of the second component Wong listed—supporting and bridging services for children and families—she discussed a state-level program and a county-level pilot in North Carolina. The state-level program is attempting to create the infrastructure to enhance how children, families, and individuals with IDD can access programs that can support their overall well-being, not just their health care. To accomplish this, the state launched a new Division of Child and Family Well-Being in the North Carolina Department of Health and Human Services. This division is drawing on the lessons of the COVID-19 pandemic regarding how different programs work together to serve children, and it is bringing together complementary programs from the departments that serve children and youth. The programs include those focused on nutrition; early intervention; children and youth, including those with special health care needs; and school and community mental health, including children with complex needs.

The goal of this effort, said Wong, is to meet the health, social, and educational needs of children and their families by enhancing how they can access programs. "We want to be able to coordinate those increased investments to get the most bang for the buck and also recognize that we really need to elevate the value of the teams and support those teams who are doing the hard work day-in and day-out," she said.

The CMS-funded, county-level North Carolina Integrated Care for Kids pilot program aims to integrate holistic care that goes beyond attending to physical and behavioral health and addresses social and educational factors for Medicaid-insured children from birth to age 20. Over the past 2 years, Wong and her colleagues have been thinking about what a blue-sky model would be for children, including those with IDD, and working to get stakeholder buy-in to enact the model, which was scheduled to start in January 2022.

The pilot first uses the state's integrated, cross-sector data to identify children who need or would likely benefit from additional supports, assigning them to a family navigator who will serve as their care manager. The family meets with the family navigator to form an integrated care team of trusted individuals from across sectors, which can include a school counselor, neighbor, or peer. Together, the family, navigator, and care team collaborate to create a shared action plan, which is something the families wanted to ensure that everyone on the care team is clear about the individual's and family's goals. The family and family navigator meet at least quarterly to discuss unmet or emerging needs.

In terms of investing in what matters to individuals with IDD, the key is to link payments to measures of whole-person well-being. This is different from the current status, wherein payers and health systems track measures that focus on health care utilization, such as the percentage of children getting well-child visits or immunizations. Meaningful and more holistic performance measures would include those that assess social drivers of health, including food insecurity, housing instability, and readiness for kindergarten. They would also include quality-of-life measures, particularly for children with IDD, that assess autonomy, a sense of belonging, and life satisfaction. Alternative payment models, said Wong, should offer the flexibility providers in the holistic sense need to support whole-person care and meet individuals' changing needs. It is important, too, that the payment models have a person-centered design with broad stakeholder engagement and shared governance. They should include new "cost of health" measures that focus on a longer time horizon to incentivize prevention and care over a lifetime, measure across sectors to solve the "wrong pocket" problem, and address the whole family to incentivize multigenerational approaches.

Discussion

An audience member commented that the electronic health record makes it almost impossible to think about the type of care coordination the panelists discussed and wondered if the panelists had any thoughts or had seen pilot programs on transforming electronic health records so they could gather information from different sectors. Lewis replied that one challenge is that electronic health records are still not interoperable even across health systems, let alone across other sectors. She noted that Medicaid systems, particularly home- and community-based agencies, are considering significant investments in modernizing their electronic record systems with American Rescue Plan Act funds, which might produce savings by reducing the tremendous amount of time and resources moving paper around entities outside of the health care system.

Kitzhaber commented that before spending more money on electronic health records, the community should step back and think about what information the individual needs to be at the center of care and build an electronic record that supports that need rather than trying to fit it into the current version. He also remarked that while health care systems should not be responsible for schools, housing, or social services that are not their core competencies, they do have a responsibility to bend the cost curve so that the 25 cents on the health care dollar that does not contribute to health can fund the resources needed to address the social determinants of health.

Wong noted that the county-level pilot program hired an external vendor to create and run an integrated care platform. Families can designate role-based access to neighbors, teachers, and anyone else who provides support for their children. Ayers thought that was a great way to provide autonomy to families.

Ayers then asked the panelists for ways beyond driving coordination that can include consumers in their care and enable them to influence the system. Kitzhaber replied that that would require designing a system that intentionally creates a space for consumers to be engaged rather than treating them as an afterthought. Lewis commented that the DD Act has funded entities nationwide that create a formal table for person-centered engagement for the IDD community. These councils provide the opportunity to formalize person-centered systems and structures, include peer-based options in models of coordinated care, and allow adults with IDD to continue to control their own lives, make decisions, maintain their legal rights, and get additional support for communication and decision making. Wong added that it is important for not just adults but also young people to have a seat on those councils.

SPOTLIGHT PRESENTATION: SPECIALIZED TELEMEDICINE FOR INDIVIDUALS WITH IDD

In the third spotlight presentation, Trivedi (StationMD) commented that he and his collaborators founded their physician practice based on their own experiences of seeing individuals with IDD come to the ED and urgent care for reasons that did not warrant that level of care. StationMD provides telemedicine-based care for approximately 35,000 individuals in 13 states. All of its physicians are board certified and go through a specialized curriculum and training to understand the needs of the IDD population, including its nonclinical factors. He noted that he used to be one of those physicians who had never received such training. Staff members conduct thousands of virtual encounters annually with individuals with IDD and monthly peer reviews to get to know the needs of this population, the needs of the family members, and the needs of the ecosystem in which they live.

Over the nearly 7 years that Trivedi has been doing this work, he has noticed that providing a virtual platform for individuals with IDD and their families has reduced the stress and logistical challenges that used to arise from having to go to the ED for things as simple as a medication refill. The virtual platform has also produced predictability and reliability in terms of always having a physician trained in the special needs of this population and independence that has allowed individuals with IDD to continue living in the community. In addition, the StationMD system has reduced staff overtime and turnover among group home and support services providers and medical costs for insurers. Data from its clients show an average of 85 percent treat-in-place rate, reducing ED and urgent care transfers.

In addition to providing medical care, StationMD provides help and care integration. He and his colleagues completed a project with the Missouri Division of Mental Health to build an interoperable system that includes electronic data from LTSS providers, physicians, and primary care. This enables him, when he evaluates someone, to see what their life and work goals are and what their home setting is like.

TECHNICAL AND POLICY OPPORTUNITIES IN FINANCING AND PAYMENT

In the penultimate session, four panelists discussed the type of technical work and policy changes needed to improve financing and payment and enable the innovative, high-quality models of care for people with IDD that previous speakers throughout the workshop discussed. The panelists were Alyna Chien (Boston Children's Hospital), Colleen Kidney (Human Services Research Institute), Joan Alker (Georgetown McCourt School of Public

Policy), and Joshua Sharfstein (Johns Hopkins Bloomberg School of Public Health). Following the presentations, Julia Bascom (Autistic Self Advocacy Network) moderated an open discussion.

Risk Adjustment for Payment of Health and HCBS

Colleagues Chien and Kidney first provided their perspective on people with disabilities. Quoting the 2006 United Nations Convention on the Rights of Persons with Disabilities, Kidney said that "persons with disabilities include those who have long-term physical, mental, intellectual, or sensory impairments which in interaction with various barriers may hinder their full and effective participation in society on an equal basis with others." This statement, she said, acknowledges that disability is the interaction between the individual and the environment, as opposed to thinking of it as a medical condition to be cured or avoided. "This societal perspective challenges us to think about how inclusive environments and communities may lessen challenges experienced by people with disabilities," said Kidney. It is from this perspective, said Chien, that she and Kidney think about challenges and solutions for payers, payment incentives, and risk adjustment.

Ideally, said Chien, payment and risk adjustment design for people with IDD would begin with some understanding of the full size of the population and the levels of functional ability within it. Instead, they work with a situation in which IDD prevalence is 2.6–12.3 percent of the national population, depending on data sources and methods, which corresponds to 28.6–38.7 million individuals. She added that the IDD population is underestimated in both the health care and HCBS sectors. For example, claims-based algorithms that do not have a disability or IDD lens can miss about 20 percent of people with IDD.

Out of the total IDD population, some 5.0–5.6 million individuals have the highest levels of need. However, said Kidney, HCBS likely falls short of serving all of those high-need individuals. In 2017, some 807,000 people were receiving HCBS through Medicaid waivers, with another 200,000 on the wait list. "There is clearly a gap to be explored to ensure more individuals receive the supports and care they need, and better payment is one way to help close that gap," said Kidney.

Even though health care administrative databases or existing HCBS are not identifying everyone with IDD, estimates suggest that spending on this population is in the range of $500 million annually. Adding in societal costs, such as parental leave time or work loss, increases this estimate to $500 billion, said Chien. "With high spending and suboptimal quality processes and outcomes that were well covered in every other presentation before ours, and a concern about how equitable service delivery is, it is definitely worthwhile to examine the effectiveness of health care and home and community-based services for people with IDD," said Chien. She added that thinking about this as a joint problem for health care and HCBS to solve makes sense given the numerous studies supporting the idea that HCBS spending reduces health care utilization.

After Kidney's reminder that financing is how dollars get into the system and payment is how money goes to individuals for their services or to payers to provide those services, Chien explained that risk adjustment occurs within a context of an overall payment strategy. In particular, it applies to a strategy also known as "capitation" or "managed care" that aims to give providers a set amount for beneficiaries irrespective of whether they present for care. The idea is that this strategy is important for work that is complex and difficult to otherwise quantify and for limiting unnecessary spending. She offered that it can occur without a quality improvement or pay-for-performance incentive. However, both can be blended with quality improvement or pay-for-performance to create one form of value-based care.

Risk adjustment, said Chien, is a statistical method that accounts for how characteristics of a given population may relate to an outcome, which in this case is usually annual spending. It is critical for rewarding those providing insurance or health care or HCBS to patients who are more complex over less complex ones, because if the payment level is not right, cherry-picking or adverse selection occurs. The inputs to risk adjustment, she explained, usually cover just three characteristics: age, sex, and the diagnostic costs accumulated over time, often a year.

In health care, risk adjustment performs modestly, noted Chien, as calculated by what is known as R-squared, where a value of 1 is perfect and 0 is no value provided. For both health care and HCBS, R-squared is 0.1–0.25. Risk adjustment can be improved in many ways, but the most critical features of optimizing it for payment are to articulate programmatic goals and define and measure care quality and outcomes, said Chien. Doing so can raise R-squared to 0.3–0.5, and this is what the workshop's presentations have tried to do.

Making the invisible visible can make risk adjustment better, said Chien. Despite the many ways to identify individuals with IDD from diagnostic information, adding in HCBS data might do a better job. For example, she would like to see if individuals who qualify for HCBS in health care risk adjustment models are actually receiving those services. Kidney added that it is important to consider and measure care quality and outcomes to improve risk adjustment, as is knowing the programmatic goals and overall budget before addressing risk adjustment. The latter will likely lead to tough conversations about who will be eligible for services and what they will receive, said Kidney. "The more concrete and measurable the goals are, the more precise risk adjustment can be," she said. Chien ended the presentation by noting that it is important to run experiments to test risk adjustment and involve stakeholders as much as possible in the process.

Financing Care Systems for People with IDD

Some 13.9 million children have special health care needs, including those with IDD, said Alker. Private insurance covers 51 percent, and Medicaid and the Children's Health Insurance Program (CHIP) cover another 36 percent of those children. She noted that Medicaid does not require that a child be uninsured to be eligible for coverage, but CHIP does. Medicaid can act as a wraparound to private employer coverage that may not meet a child's needs. Approximately 10 percent of these children with special health care needs have a gap in coverage. In a blue-sky world, Alker would love to ignore coverage and just think about outcomes and quality of care, but unfortunately, she said, insurance is a price of admission to the U.S. health care system, which means worrying about coverage.

Data from the congressionally chartered Medicaid and CHIP Payment and Access Commission shows that children with autism or developmental delay are more likely to be covered by Medicaid or CHIP, while children with an intellectual disability are more than twice as likely to be in Medicaid or CHIP. She explained that though Medicaid is a federal-state program, the states are in charge of designing their delivery systems and systems of care. This means that the states are the place to start to reconceptualize public financing of health care, given that Medicaid is by far the largest payer of the public financing system. She also noted that Medicaid offers a fair amount of flexibility even without waivers.

Multiple types of waivers exist, with Section 1115 demonstration waivers providing the broadest Medicaid authority. Their name derives from Section 1115 of the Social Security Act, which allows the HHS Secretary to grant waivers of certain requirements in Medicaid or CHIP or to spend and receive federal funds in different ways, although the federal matching rate cannot be waived. These waivers must be necessary to conduct a true health coverage demonstration, experiment, or pilot project and promote the objectives of Medicaid (to provide comprehensive health insurance coverage to primarily, though not exclusively, to low-income people).

Waivers, explained Alker, should only last for the period necessary to carry out the experiment or demonstration. The initial approval period is usually 5 years, with 3-year or 5-year (if dual eligibles are included) renewals or extensions. During the Trump administration, CMS authorized 10-year extensions to political allies in Florida, Texas, and Tennessee, which Alker said did not comport with the statute. Waivers can also go too far, she added, such as the Trump administration's approval to impose work requirements, which federal courts have struck down.

Administrations from both political parties have decided that demonstrations must be "budget neutral" for the federal government, though this is not a statutory requirement. Alker explained that budget neutrality is a hypothetical construct. She encouraged any program seeking a waiver to think creatively about it and not let it get in the way of initially considering reforms.

Alker said that the Affordable Care Act added the requirement for a public comment period before CMS can grant a Section 1115 waiver. She believes this is great because it forces states to take comments, think about them, and hopefully make changes before submitting their application to CMS. In fact, states have to explain how they have responded to the comments.

A Population Health Framework for Caring for Individuals with IDD

Starting with the big picture, Sharfstein said that the core focus of the system of care for people with IDD should be on the goals that they have for themselves, for their health and well-being. At the same time, the goal from the systems perspective should be to improve the health of the entire population of people with disabilities while also helping each individual meet their goals. State agencies, he added, have opportunities to monitor population health, develop strategies for health improvement, and mobilize community providers, health insurers, and clinical providers to implement them.

The elements of the public health framework are assessment, policy development, and assurance. "First, you look at where things are, then you figure out how to make them better through different policies, and then you see whether that works or not," explained Sharfstein. For the assessment piece, state agencies should be able to answer questions about how often people are hospitalized or readmitted quickly after discharge, the rates of preventable illness and death, and the percentage of people receiving recommended preventive health care, such as vaccines. Clinical providers, health insurers, and community providers can then analyze these data to determine why one managed care organization is able to deliver vaccines while another is not, for example, or why one is seeing much higher levels of preventable illness than another.

"Once you have an assessment of where things are and you understand the picture in different categories, then you can make strategies," said Sharfstein. "That is the policy development part of public health." For example, if dehydration seems to be a common cause of hospital admission for a particular health system, then the system can implement policies and actions to prevent dehydration for people at high risk. Similarly, if one particular health plan is seeing higher rates of readmission, a review may be appropriate to understand why and what preventive steps that health plan can put in place to address that problem. If a particular individual or group of individuals seems to be going in and out of the hospital frequently, a case manager can see if additional services may be needed or identify other issues.

Regarding assurance, state agencies can use data to understand the role of different systems in supporting greater health for people with developmental disabilities. Data, said Sharfstein, are a tool for measurement, oversight, and accountability, and they can also identify of how states can help people with IDD stay healthy and achieve their goals.

Discussion

Bascom opened the discussion with a question from the audience, which wondered where the early and periodic screening, diagnostic, and treatment (EPSDT) benefit for children under age 21 who are enrolled in Medicaid[17] fits into the continuum of services given that some states should cover many of the benefits in HCBS under EPSDT. Alker responded that in her view, EPSDT should never be waived, though it has been in one state. Nevertheless, Alker identified a lack of understanding about what the EPSDT benefit is and how rich it should be, so the way states actualize this benefit varies greatly. She noted that CMS may be working to develop a more consistent definition to reduce that variability. Sharfstein added that Medicaid's concept of EPSDT differs from the pediatric benefit from private insurance, and he worries that as children go into private insurance, they could lose some important benefits. EPSDT, he explained, creates an expectation that states will meet the needs of children, as opposed to private insurance's approach of covering an enumerated list of services.

Another question on EPSDT asked the panelists to speak about the role of medical necessity in determining what a state's Medicaid program will cover in terms of HCBS. Alker replied she thinks about EPSDT as being broader than private insurance definitions of medical necessity. Theoretically, she said, any issue that screening identifies, including developmental delays, should be treated, period. She noted that the EPSDT benefit lacks the arbitrary limits of private insurance, which provides more opportunities to think creatively about providing care for someone with IDD. Sharfstein added that it is hard to imagine that this benefit could expand to include the entire HCBS waiver program, as much as that would help individuals with IDD.

Bascom asked the panelists for their ideas on how the government can get private insurers to contribute to financing HCBS, particularly in the context that Medicaid does not cover many individuals of all ages with IDD. Chien responded that autism activism has been moving the needle, with many

---

[17] Additional information is available at https://www.medicaid.gov/medicaid/benefits/early-and-periodic-screening-diagnostic-and-treatment/index.html (accessed April 28, 2022).

self-insured employer plans now including autism services as an automatic benefit. The only problem here, said Bascom, is that many insurance plans only cover very specific types of services for autism rather than coverage based on what individuals need. Alker added that states are the locus for regulating private insurers, making it unlikely that the federal government will take action on this issue anytime soon.

The next question asked the panelists to discuss how Section 1115 waivers could help build person-directed, holistic coordination. Alker said the place to start is to identify the barriers that a waiver would overcome, though she cautioned that Medicaid will be unable to become the payer to address all the inadequacies in the social safety net, such as inadequate housing.

Responding to a question about how self-determination could be structured under the HCBS benefit to promote health equity, Sharfstein replied that even though individuals are making decisions, it should be possible to ensure that the services provided are appropriate, fair, and actually helping people who might be the most likely to have the greatest needs. Achieving that requires designing a self-directed program that considers all the types of services a group of people might need, trains beneficiaries as to how to make the best use of self-direction, and then aggregates data to make sure that people are getting the benefits they need in a way that narrows rather than expands gaps.

Chien added that it is important to define what health equity means, given the wide range of abilities across the IDD population, and think about whether it is more important to society to care for those with the greatest need or if equity means providing some services to everybody regardless of need. In her opinion, it might be easier to be fair and equitable across a narrow band of need than to figure out what is equitable across a wider range. Kidney noted that collecting and analyzing data is fundamental to addressing this issue. Alker commented that she and her colleagues have been encouraging the Biden administration to require an equity analysis in a waiver application.

SCALING WORKFORCE SOLUTIONS

The final session explored what needs to happen to prepare as many clinicians as possible to care for individuals with IDD. The three panelists were Helen Burstin (Council of Medical Specialty Societies), Karrie Shogren (Kansas University Center on Developmental Disabilities, University of Kansas), and Andrés Gallegos (National Council on Disability [NCD]). Sandra Schnieder (American College of Emergency Physicians) moderated a discussion period.

The Role of Professional Organizations in Moving the Field Forward

Burstin's organization represents 47 primary care and specialty societies covering the entire breadth of medicine, which is relevant because many individuals with IDD interact with a wide range of primary care providers and specialists, she explained. In terms of thinking about operationalizing how professional organizations can move the field and accelerate change, she offered examples of opportunities to think big, starting with capitalizing on lessons from the COVID-19 pandemic. "In terms of cross-specialty, cross-disciplinary collaboration, we have seen levels of collaboration and speed with rigor in ways we have never seen before," said Burstin.

For example, specialty societies developed cross-specialty guidelines in weeks to months, instead of the usual years. Burstin said that they quickly stood up resource centers and shared information, tools, and training. In particular, she commended the American College of Emergency Physicians for issuing field guides with wide reach for easy reference and in multiple languages. "If we can do this for something like COVID, we can work more closely for something like ensuring high-quality care for patients and families of those with IDD," she said.

Another example was the cross-professional collaboration spearheaded by the National Academies of Medicine Action Collaborative on Countering the U.S. Opioid Epidemic. Burstin called this a remarkable public–private partnership, and she noted the speed with which it has developed a core competency domain for opioid education based on core knowledge, collaboration, and clinical practice. She added that much of that work could be broadly applicable to developing core competencies and domains to care effectively for patients and families with IDD. Similarly, the collaborative has been developing a patient-centered chronic pain journey map that can help individuals think through where they are along that journey, and she wondered if the IDD community could build such a patient journey map for neurodiverse individuals. That might help health care understand what this journey looks like and then build the resources that would help individuals and their families traverse it.

Turning to the subject of the health information technology infrastructure and electronic health records, Burstin noted that the IDD population experiences a tremendous amount of fragmented care across multiple entities in and outside of health care. She wondered if it would be possible to take an inclusive, patient- and family-centered view of interoperability for the IDD community. This would entail identifying the resources that clinicians, patients, and their caregivers need at their fingertips to ensure the best care possible. "What is that quick information that should always be available on all patients regardless of where they are being seen that would make a difference?" she asked, suggesting that this should include the social determinants of health.

Burstin noted that decades of experience show that a general "rising tide lifts all boats" philosophy will not eliminate disparities. "We have to do something targeted," she said. She quoted Albert Einstein: "We cannot solve our problems with the same thinking we used when we created them." She called on the community to think big, break down silos, and think about how to work together with the speed and efficiency that the IDD population demands.

Disrupting the Systemic Barriers and Biases That Limit Options for Individuals with IDD

Shogren noted that the work on systemic collaboration and self-determination she would speak about has been led, shaped, and driven by advocates with IDD who are continuously pushing for systems and supporters in them to recognize their self-determination. She also commented that community-engaged, participatory research, policy, and practice are critical components for achieving the advances needed to support individuals with IDD.

Shogren said that three things are essential to moving toward a future where systems and supports are integrated in ways that advance equity, diversity, and inclusion. The first is the need to acknowledge that systems are complex, which makes systemic collaboration that cuts across all systems that affect the lives of people with IDD essential to disrupt the barriers and biases that limit their options. However, the current system places the burden of integrating the systems intended to provide those supports on individuals and their families, which perpetuates inequity and represents a failure of systems, said Shogren.

In her view, systems need to be built in ways that foster systemic collaboration by facilitating better cross-system navigation and integration, having navigators that carry information across systems, and implementing data systems that facilitate communication and information sharing and eliminate duplication. Each system, be it education, health, or community-based services and supports, is less effective in isolation, said Shogren. However, fighting for systemic collaboration should not be required of people with IDD and their families. Rather, systems and their leaders need to be the ones breaking down barriers, eliminating bias, and working to build a new transdisciplinary system.

The second thing needed to move to a better system is to recognize that within complex systems, people with disabilities have the right to self-determine their own lives with effective supports. While everyone needs supports to engage in life and community, people with IDD need personalized supports that enable them to engage in the systems they choose in the way they choose.

The third thing needed is for people with disabilities to be involved in identifying the characteristics and collaborations across the systems that support them. In other words, said Shogren, they must be empowered to shape their own care and how care systems are organized to facilitate systemic collaboration. "All too often, we fail to provide these supports in self-determined ways, limiting opportunities," she said.

Citing language from the DD Act, Shogren said, "disability is a natural part of the human experience that does not diminish the right of individuals with developmental disabilities to live independently, to exert choice and control, and to fully participate in and contribute to their communities through full integration and inclusion in the economic, political, social, cultural, and educational mainstream of U.S. society." Similar language, she said, is included in all disability rights laws and international treaties. However, it is critical to instantiate these values into systems as they are disrupted. All too often, care and support systems fail to view people with disabilities as full partners in designing systems for systemic collaboration or self-determining their personalized supports.

People with disabilities, said Shogren, have the same right as everyone else to make decisions and inform changes that affect them, which reflects the adage "nothing about us without us." "I think a blue-sky future must recognize our responsibility to make this a reality and not only view people with intellectual and developmental disabilities as recipients of care systems but instead as full partners in their implementation and design," she said. While research shows that promoting engagement and self-determination leads to better outcomes across systems, barriers and bias limit this opportunity and marginalize people with IDD, particularly those with intersectional identities and complex needs.

Pushing even further, Shogren said that people with IDD have the right to lead workforce solutions. "We need to consider how people with intellectual and developmental disabilities cannot only be recipients of changes but also leaders," she said. "We have an opportunity to consider new and different career pathways for people with intellectual and developmental disabilities as we integrate systems." The challenge, she noted, is to leverage lived experience to design integrated systems and create new expectations and opportunities for employment, leadership, and professional roles for people with IDD who have the knowledge and interest to take on these roles and advance change.

Shogren recalled one young person with IDD who participated in a randomized trial on effective interventions to support self-determination during movement from school-based systems to adult community-based supports and services. The trial involved training educators to deliver the interventions that would enable students to set self-directed goals based on a future they envisioned and thus grow in their self-determination. This student challenged

Shogren and her collaborators by saying he wanted to be the coach or instructor. He wanted to deliver the intervention and support others with disabilities because he could share his experiences and advocate with them.

This comment forced her to ask herself why she had not thought of that. "Why had we not broken down barriers and created opportunities for people with intellectual and developmental disabilities to be co-trained as professional facilitators and collaborate with other professionals?" she asked. "It was a failure in vision that this young man brought to our attention." Today, she and her colleagues are working to make that vision a reality. They are finding pathways to support people with IDD who are interested in such a career and for them to partner with educators and other disability support providers to deliver interventions.

Shogren asked everyone to consider how they can work to remove barriers and build integrated systems across health, clinical care, education, and community supports and to think about approaches that will support people with IDD to lead change and leverage their lived experiences to create a better future for themselves, their peers, and all of society.

Potential Federal Policy Opportunities

The NCD, explained Gallegos, is an independent federal agency charged with advising the president, the administration, Congress, and federal agencies on all policy matters affecting people with disabilities in the United States and its territories. He noted, as speakers on the workshop's first day did, that medical schools do not provide a meaningful education in treating patients with disabilities, and graduates enter residency and fellowship programs with little or no skills, knowledge, comfort, confidence, or awareness in the proper treatment. These deficits, he said, are reflected in adverse outcomes. Moreover, while LCME and the Accreditation Council on Graduate Medical Education (ACGME) have done little to develop providers who can offer culturally competent and appropriate care to millions of individuals with disabilities. Gallegos said the federal government can play an important role in doing so.

Section 5307 of the Affordable Care Act requires the HHS Secretary to collaborate with experts in minority health, cultural competency, and prevention and with organizations such as health professional societies, licensing and accreditation entities, health professional schools, public health disability groups, community-based organizations, and others as deemed appropriate by the Secretary to develop model disability cultural competency curricula and then to disseminate those curricula through an Internet clearinghouse. This, said Gallegos, was never done, and the NCD is pushing for it. "We have been working on a health equity framework for people across all categories of disabilities, and the development of a disability cultural competency curricula is one of our four core components of that framework," he said. However, added Gallegos, Section 5307 does not go far enough because it does not mandate adoption of such a curriculum as part of every medical, dental, nursing, and other health professional training program, including residencies and fellowships.

The other three core components of this framework are enhanced and deliberate data capturing, adopting the U.S. Access Board's standards on medical diagnostic equipment as binding regulations, and designating people with disabilities as a medically underserved population under the Public Health Service Act. This last component, said Gallegos, is essential because it would enable them to obtain the associated benefits, including federal funding for health centers and public health infrastructure, such as FQHCs, eligibility to apply for federal funding to develop and operate community health centers, access to loan repayment and training programs in the Health Resources and Services Administration workforce development and training programs, incentives for physicians to treat the designated population (via higher Medicare and Medicaid reimbursement rates), and preferences for research at federal agencies, including the National Institutes of Health.

Typically, said Gallegos, the medically underserved designation requires population grouping based on geography, which is not applicable for people with disabilities. Therefore, Congress will have to revise Section 330 of the Public Health Service Act. Absent that, the next approach would be to designate people with disabilities as a health disparities population under the Minority Health and Health Disparities Research and Education Act of 2000, which would provide substantially similar benefits to those provided by the medically underserved population designation, he explained. Gallegos noted that Congress is once again considering the HEADs Up Act, which would designate people with IDD as a medically underserved population.

If those efforts fail, the fallback position is to tackle the problem piecemeal, which would include securing loan forgiveness programs that would recruit providers to dedicate their professional lives for the care of people with disabilities, making significant investments in research to address their health disparities, and securing higher Medicare and Medicaid reimbursement for the additional time that providers spend caring for this population. A piecemeal effort would also include instituting federal grants to fund recruiting people with disabilities into health professions and health management. "The issues plaguing the workforce and the ableism that we see in health care and that was brought to light during the pandemic is attributed in part to the absence of people with disabilities within the health care workforce and … in C-suites of health care systems, hospitals, and their boards," said Gallegos.

Other policy opportunities include strengthening Section 503 of the Rehabilitation Act of 1973, which prohibits disability-based discrimination by federal contractors and calls for them to implement affirmative action in hiring people with disabilities, with an aspirational goal of increasing participation by 7 percent. Hospitals and health care systems are rarely challenged to meet that requirement, said Gallegos. "There is significant room to improve those regulations to help push health care systems to hiring people with disabilities and to foster a more welcoming environment so that current workforce feels comfortable in self-identifying their own disabilities," he said.

If "carrots," or incentives, are not sufficient to develop a culturally competent and more welcoming workforce for people with disabilities in general and IDD specifically, then it is time to turn to a "sharper stick," or disincentive, said Gallegos. That would involve invoking Section 504 of the Rehabilitation Act of 1973, which prohibits disability-based discrimination by recipients of federal financial assistance and holds hospitals and health care systems accountable for not providing culturally competent care for people with disabilities in general and people with IDD in particular. The problem with both regulations is that they lack specificity, making them difficult to enforce. However, the HHS Office for Civil Rights, which has primary jurisdiction and responsibility for enforcing Section 504 with respect to health care providers, will be unveiling its notice of proposed rulemaking to strengthen the regulations in the first quarter of 2022. "If we cannot address the affective domain of learning and cannot achieve a change of heart, then let us tame them by more detailed requirements and more robust enforcement," said Gallegos.

He commented on the significant and meaningful federal opportunity to fully and permanently fund HCBS beyond the $150 billion in the Medicaid program. The goal would be to provide permanent and enhanced funding to offer Medicaid matching funds for HCBS if states choose to participate and meet certain requirements, said Gallegos.

Discussion

Schneider opened by asking Shogren how she would enable all the service providers who care for an individual with IDD to know what every other one is doing. Shogren replied that the most important step would be to empower and incentivize cross-system communications. "The inability to move basic information from health systems to community-based systems, from education systems to others, is a limiting factor. It requires that mothers, fathers, families, and people with disabilities to be the ones that are stewards of all that information," she said, "of course, they want to be stewards of that process, but they should not bear all of that responsibility." Integrating systems and providing mechanisms for doing so is essential, she added.

Burstin agreed and noted how difficult it is even for different parts of the medical system to communicate and share information. She would like to see efforts to improve interoperability across health systems broadened to include interoperability across all the systems that care for individuals with IDD.

Schneider asked Burstin for her ideas on how to integrate the items that Gallegos discussed into the medical school curriculum, particularly bringing more people with disabilities into the system. Burstin replied that it is important to both help trainees understand the rest of the world and bring the rest of the world into their classes. For example, work that her organization is doing with ACGME on equity includes having a physician with a disability talk about his experiences of going through medical school in a wheelchair. She also stressed the importance of altering the medical profession's overwhelming perception that the quality of life for individuals with IDD is so much worse than for the general population. Gallegos added that while many medical schools are starting to form panels of people with disabilities who will speak to students, that is not enough. "You need a full, robust curriculum," he said. "You need to have dedicated time within the curriculum to get in depth on these topics and not just have a cursory introductory or a presentation over lunch to fill this void."

An audience member commented that dentistry has standards that would meet Section 504 requirements, to which Gallegos replied that the NCD pushed dentistry to adopt standards, something that has not succeeded so far with medical education. In fact, he questioned whether new 504 regulations will push hard enough to address curriculum and accreditation issues. He did note that the council is discussing with the Joint Commission and CMS the idea that Joint Commission surveys should include disability care and disability cultural competency in their checklist. The council is also imploring the Joint Commission to include people with disabilities on its survey teams.

Given the wide range of community service providers involved in caring for individuals with IDD, Schneider asked Shogren if it is even possible to integrate them all and how that could be accomplished beyond assembling them in a room and giving a 1-hour show-and-tell presentation. Shogren replied that moving beyond such a presentation is critical, even for medical provider training, which will require pushing to have people with disabilities included in these organizations, not just speaking to them once in a while. Burstin commented that the meaningful use funds that incentivized the medical community to adopt electronic health records should extend to community-based organizations so that they have the resources to implement those systems. She also promoted the idea of getting medical students, residents, and practicing doctors outside of the walls of the health system and into the community, rather than bringing the community to the medical system.

Schneider asked the panelists for one or two major strategies for the workforce. Burstin said that if she had a magic wand, she would implement a process to develop uniform, collaborative standards of care for individuals with

IDD across all specialties, with input from individuals with IDD and their families. Shogren said she wants to figure out how to create seats at the table for all members of the IDD community that are equally valued and respected. This would involve supporting them so they can be part of the process and recognizing that failing to listen to them and their families is preventing the system from building on their experiences to drive change. Gallegos said he wants Congress to designate all people with disabilities as a medically underserved population and the HHS Secretary to develop a model curriculum and make it mandatory.

Commenting from her perspective as an ED physician, Schneider noted that almost every day, a group comes to her and says its members are special and the ED needs to change. While acknowledging that EDs do need to change how they deal with individuals with certain needs, she and her colleagues only have so much bandwidth. "How can we bring this together so that we are not reacting to each group, because if I go out and wave the flag for IDD, which I would, there is going to be somebody else handing me another flag 10 minutes later?" she asked. She wondered if the panelists had any thoughts about strategies she could use to implement change more broadly. Shogren said that those battles will persist as long as systems are building segmented solutions for different groups. The challenge, she said, is to use the principles of universal design to build a system that supports all people and then add increasingly specialized supports and services with it. Gallegos did not have an answer but did note the intersectionality between those other groups vying for attention and the disability community.

CLOSING COMMENTS DAY THREE

Gilfillan provided his take on the workshop from his perspective as a family clinician who cared for a large population of individuals with IDD, a former health insurance executive, and the first director of the CMS Innovation Center. He noted the tremendous progress from 35 years ago, when he cared for some 400 adult men with IDD. Much of that progress, he said, is the result of the advocacy efforts of individuals, families, and the organizations they created. "It is really a remarkable story of what dedicated volunteers can do over a long period of time, and it is impressive," said Gilfillan.

One of his takeaways was that many excellent models of care exist for individuals with IDD, but they are not scalable because the system is not in a position to support scaling. Adequate knowledge, know-how, and commitment are available, along with a workforce, one that is not as well trained as everyone would like but that families and individuals with IDD appreciate greatly, Gillfillan said. Approaches to training and extending that workforce exist. What is missing, he emphasized, is a unified approach on the finance and payment side. Instead, that system is fragmented and fundamentally inadequate; as Kitzhaber pointed out, it probably has enough money, but it is not apportioning that money so as to make a difference.

Despite the progress he has seen, the population of individuals with IDD is still behind the general population in the most basic measures of health, life expectancy, chronic disease incidence, and outcomes. He noted the almost one million people on a wait list for LTSS, the only wait list for health care services in the United States. "We have the services and know how to provide those services, but we as a society have decided not to do that yet," said Gilfillan.

The health care system is a small but significant part of the problem, he said. Individuals with IDD have the same difficulties dealing with it as others do because it is not set up to be supportive and provide ongoing, continuous, integrated care. A bigger part is the failure of the nation to go upstream in terms of the drivers of health care and recognize the effects that IDD has on population health as a whole. Making health care better requires making the IDD population visible. "We need to define it and understand it," said Gilfillan. It is important for the public to understand the population's size, conditions, and outcomes. The nation also needs to address workforce issues, build models of integration, and demand that health systems engage actively in developing integrated and coordinated systems for this population.

Ultimately, said Gilfillan, the nation needs a community-based system of care, though he did not have an answer about the necessary accountable party. He noted that providers' clinical perspective is not aligned well with the perspective needed to support the IDD population, but providers are in the community and connected to and trusted by those individuals. "I would think that we should think real hard about whether or not we should build an accountable entity around health systems," he said. He offered that the Robert Wood Johnson Foundation's Raising the Bar initiative has developed creative principles for how health systems can work with community-based organizations, which he thought could be worth exploring as a possible approach to engaging providers.

His final comments addressed the rethinking at the national level about the nature of the safety net for individuals and how health systems and the nation can address the social determinants of health. "We need to think about how the IDD community fits into that broader issue of addressing a more just society," said Gilfillan. He suggested setting the stage for the general public and policy makers to learn more about ableism. "As we talk about structural racism, as we talk about the economic determinants of health, we need to also talk about the realities of ableism that underlie so much of the discrimination against the population that we talked about over these last several days," he said. "If we are really going to address all those solutions to improve health to this population, we need to find a voice that is both specific at addressing those needs, but we also have to align with these broader forces that are pushing for a social service system that provides a fair opportunity to achieve optimal health broadly defined as individuals for all people."

The United States has enormous resources, but they are not distributed in ways that allow for individuals to fully achieve their goals in life and optimal development of health, he said. He would like to see a coalition that would bring together the different voices in the IDD community and align them with the broader efforts toward more social justice and creating a better safety net system that addresses the social determinants of health. "That may be an important next step for this community as we consider the outcomes from this meeting," said Gilfillan.

Hoangmai Pham said that the very best National Academies workshops lead to action. "We hope that after you leave, you stay connected with us and with each other and take inspiration from these conversations to make change for the IDD community," said Pham. With that, the workshop adjourned.

References

ADHCE (Alliance for Disability in Health Care Education). 2019. *Core competencies on disability for health care education.* Peapack, NJ: Alliance for Disability in Health Care Education.

AHRQ (Agency for Healthcare Research and Quality). 2014. *Working for quality: Achieving better health and health care for all Americans.* Washington, DC: Agency for Healthcare Research and Quality.

Bodenheimer, T., E. H. Wagner, and K. Grumbach. 2002. Improving primary care for patients with chronic illness. *Journal of the American Medical Association* 288(14):1775–1779. https://doi.org/10.1001/jama.288.15.1909.

Bowen, C. N., S. M. Havercamp, S. Karpiak Bowen, and G. Nye. 2020. A call to action: Preparing a disability-competent health care workforce. *Disability and Health Journal* 13(4):100941. https://doi.org/10.1016/j.dhjo.2020.100941.

Breslin, M. L., and S. Yee. 2009. *The current state of health care for people with disabilities.* https://files.eric.ed.gov/fulltext/ED507726.pdf (accessed August 31, 2022).

CCA (Commonwealth Care Alliance). 2019. *Commonwealth Care Alliance presentation for Vermont Blueprint Health.* https://blueprintforhealth.vermont.gov/sites/bfh/files/CCA-at-Blueprint-for-Health-VT-vFinal.pdf (accessed May 25, 2022).

CCA. 2021. *CCA annual report: 2020.* https://www.commonwealthcarealliance.org/about-us/newsroom-publications/2021-cca-annual-report (accessed May 25, 2022).

Crane, J. M., J. G. Strickler, A. T. Lash, A. Macerollo, J. A. Prokup, K. A. Rich, A. C. Robinson, C. N. Whalen Smith, and S. M. Havercamp. 2021. Getting comfortable with disability: The short- and long-term effects of a clinical encounter. *Disability and Health Journal* 14(2):100993.

Ennis, G., and M. Tofa. 2020. Collective impact: A review of the peer-reviewed research. *Australian Social Work* 73(1):32–47. https://doi.org/10.1080/0312407X.2019.1602662.

Family Voices. n.d. *About Family Voices*. https://familyvoices.org/about (accessed May 25, 2022).

Fulmer, T., E. Flaherty, and K. Hyer. 2004. The geriatric interdisciplinary team training (GITT) program. *Gerontology and Geriatrics Education* 24(2):3–12. https://doi.org/10.1300/j021v24n02_02.

Havercamp, S. M., W. R. Barnhart, A. C. Robinson, and C. N. Whalen Smith. 2021. What should we teach about disability? National consensus on disability competencies for health care education. *Disability and Health Journal* 14(2):100989. https://doi.org/10.1016/j.dhjo.2020.100989.

ICS (Independence Care System). 2016. *A blueprint for improving access to primary care for adults with physical disabilities*. https://nyhealthfoundation.org/resource/blueprint-for-improving-access-to-primary-care-adults-physical-disabilities (accessed June 15, 2022).

Iezzoni, L. I., S. R. Rao, J. Ressalam, D. Bolcic-Jankovic, N. D. Agaronnik, K. Donelan, T. Lagu, and E. G. Campbell. 2021. Physicians' perceptions of people with disability and their health care. *Health Affairs* 40(2):297–306. https://doi.org/10.1377/hlthaff.2020.01452.

Krahn, G. L., L. Hammond, and A. Turner. 2006. A cascade of disparities: Health and health care access for people with intellectual disabilities. *Mental Retardation and Developmental Disability Research Review* 12(1):70–82. https://doi.org/10.1002/mrdd.20098.

Kripke, C., M. Giammona, A. Fox, and J. Shorter. 2011. The CART model: Organized systems of care for transition age youth and adults with developmental disabilities. *International Journal of Child and Adolescent Health* 3(4):473–477.

Larson, S. A., K. C. Lakin, L. Anderson, N. Kwak, J. H. Lee, and D. Anderson. 2001. Prevalence of mental retardation and developmental disabilities: Estimates from the 1994/1995 National Health Interview Survey disability supplements. *American Journal of Mental Retardation* 106(3):231–252.

Lulinski, A., N. T. Jorwic, E. S. Tanis, and D. Braddock. 2018. *Rebalancing of long-term supports and services for individuals with intellectual and developmental disabilities in the United States*. Boulder, CO: Coleman Institute for Cognitive Disabilities, University of Colorado. https://www. https://www.colemaninstitute.org/wp-content/uploads/2018/04/SOS-Brief-2018_2_Rebalancing.pdf (accessed May 20, 2022).

Meeks, L. M., and N. R. Jain. 2018. *Accessibility, inclusion, and action in medical education: Lived experiences of learners and physicians with disabilities*. Washington, DC: Association of American Medical Colleges. https://store.aamc.org/downloadable/download/sample/sample_id/249 (accessed May 20, 2022).

NCD (National Council on Disability). 2009. *The current state of health care for people with disabilities*. Washington, DC: National Council on Disability. https://ncd.gov/publications/2009/Sept302009#CHAPTER%202 (accessed May 20, 2022).

Ning, M., J. Daniels, J. Schwartz, K. Dunlap, P. Washington, H. Kalantarian, M. Du, and D. P. Wall. 2019. Identification and quantification of gaps in access to autism resources in the United States: An infodemiological study. *Journal of Medical Internet Research* 21(7):e13094. https://doi.org/10.2196/13094.

REFERENCES

Parish-Morris, J., R. Solórzano, V. Ravindran, V. Sazawal, S. Turnacioglu, A. Zitter, J. Miller, and J. McCleery. 2018. *Immersive virtual reality to improve police interaction skills in adolescents and adults with autism spectrum disorder: Preliminary results of a feasibility and safety trial.* Paper presented at 23rd Annual CyberPsychology, CyberTherapy, and Social Networking Conference, Gatineau, Canada.

Pynchon, T. 1973. *Gravity's rainbow.* New York: Viking Press.

Reichard, A., H. Stolzle, and M. H. Fox. 2011. Health disparities among adults with physical disabilities or cognitive limitations compared to individuals with no disabilities in the United States. *Disability and Health Journal* 4(2):59–67. https://doi.org/https://doi.org/10.1016/j.dhjo.2010.05.003.

Schor, E. L. 2019. *An almost complete list of services used by families and children with special health care needs.* Palo Alto, CA: Lucile Packard Foundation for Children's Health.

Sullivan, W. F., H. Diepstra, J. Heng, S. Ally, E. Bradley, I. Casson, B. Hennen, M. Kelly, M. Korossy, K. McNeil, D. Abells, K. Amaria, K. Boyd, M. Gemmill, E. Grier, N. Kennie-Kaulbach, M. Ketchell, J. Ladouceur, A. Lepp, Y. Lunsky, S. McMillan, U. Niel, S. Sacks, S. Shea, K. Stringer, K. Sue, and S. Witherbee. 2018. Primary care of adults with intellectual and developmental disabilities: 2018 Canadian consensus guidelines. *Canadian Family Physician* 64(4):254–279.

Turnacioglu, S., V. Sazawal, R. Solórzano, J. Parish-Morris, A. Zitter, J. Miller, J. McCleery, and V. Ravindran. 2019. The state of virtual and augmented reality therapy for autism spectrum disorder. In *Virtual and Augmented Reality in Mental Health Treatment*, edited by G. Guazzaroni. Hershey, PA: IGI Global. Pp. 118–140.

U.S. Public Health Service. 2001. *Closing the gap: A national blueprint for improving the health of individuals with mental retardation. Report of the Surgeon General's conference on health disparities and mental retardation.* Washington, DC: U.S. Public Health Service.

WHO (World Health Organization). 2011. *World report on disability.* https://www.who.int/publications/i/item/9789241564182 (accessed June 15, 2022).

WHO. 2020. *Basic documents, 49th edition (including amendments adopted up to 31 May 2019).* Geneva, Switzerland: World Health Organization.

Wilkinson, J., D. Dreyfus, M. Cerreto, and B. Bokhour. 2012. "Sometimes I feel overwhelmed": Educational needs of family physicians caring for people with intellectual disability. *Intellectual and Developmental Disabilities* 50(3):243–250.

Appendix A

Workshop Agenda

DAY ONE: CURRENT CHALLENGES

December 8, 2021 | 1:00–4:00 pm Eastern Time

1:00 pm   Introductory Remarks
                  Kimberly Knackstedt, Director of Disability Policy for the Domestic Policy Council at the White House

1:10–2:05   I. Elements and Competencies of an Integrated System of Care

                  Panelists
                  - Edward Schor, Stanford University
                  - Lisa Iezzoni, Harvard Medical School
                  - Nanfi N. Lubogo, PATH CT and Family Voices

                  Moderator
                  James Perrin, Massachusetts General Hospital for Children, Harvard Medical School

2:05–3:00	II. Challenges in Workforce Strength and Preparedness

Panelists
- Matt Holder, American Academy of Developmental Medicine and Dentistry
- Susan Havercamp, The Ohio State University Nisonger Center
- Amy Hewitt, Institute on Community Integration, University of Minnesota

Moderator
Kara Ayers, University of Cincinnati College of Medicine

3:00–3:05	~ SPOTLIGHT PRESENTATION ~

- Maura Sullivan, Operation House Call, The Arc

3:05–4:00	III. Challenges in Financing and Payment

Panelists
- Michael Monson, Altarum Institute
- Ari Ne'eman, Harvard University
- Cheryl Powell, The MITRE Corporation

Moderator
Hoangmai Pham, Institute for Exceptional Care

4:00	Workshop Adjourns

DAY TWO: CURRENT AND PROMISING INTERVENTIONS
December 10, 2021 | 1:00–4:00 pm Eastern Time

1:00 pm	Introductory Remarks & Recap of Prior Day
1:10–2:05	IV. Innovative Models of Care & Care Coordination

Panelists
- Clarissa Kripke, University of California, San Francisco, School of Medicine
- Patricia Aguayo, University of Utah Health
- Lauren Easton, Commonwealth Care Alliance

APPENDIX A   *97*

                        Moderator
                        Elizabeth Mahar, The Arc, National

2:05–2:10   ~ SPOTLIGHT PRESENTATION ~
                        • Vijay Ravindran, Floreo VR

2:10–3:05   V. Innovations in Workforce Solutions: Role of General Health Care Providers

                        Panelists
                        • Kristin Sohl, University of Missouri and ECHO Autism
                        • Lisa Howley, Association of American Medical Colleges
                        • Sarah Ailey, Rush University College of Nursing

                        Moderator
                        Susan Thompson Hingle, Southern Illinois University School of Medicine

3:05–4:00   VI. Innovations in Financing and Payment

                        Panelists
                        • Brede Eschliman, Aurerra Health
                        • Sarah Scholle, National Committee on Quality Assurance
                        • Stephanie Rasmussen, Sunflower Health Plan

                        Moderator
                        Hoangmai Pham, Institute for Exceptional Care

4:00   Workshop Adjourns

DAY THREE: LOOKING FORWARD / BLUE SKIES
December 14, 2021 | 1:00–4:00 pm Eastern Time

1:00 pm   Introductory Remarks & Recap of Prior Day

1:05–2:00   VII. A New Vision for Models of Care

Panelists
- John Kitzhaber, Former Governor of Oregon
- Sharon Lewis, Health Management Associates
- Charlene Wong, Duke University

Moderators
Kara Ayers, University of Cincinnati College of Medicine
Alicia Theresa Francesca Bazzano, Special Olympics Inc.

2:00–2:05 — SPOTLIGHT PRESENTATION —
- Maulik Trivedi, StationMD

2:05–3:00 VIII. Technical and Policy Opportunities in Financing and Payment

Panelists
- Alyna Chien (Boston Children's Hospital) and Colleen Kidney (Human Services Research Institute)
- Joan Alker, Georgetown McCourt School of Public Policy
- Joshua Sharfstein, Johns Hopkins Bloomberg School of Public Health

Moderator
Julia Bascom, Autistic Self Advocacy Network

3:00–3:55 IX. Scaling Workforce Solutions

Panelists
- Helen Burstin, Council of Medical Specialty Societies
- Karrie Shogren, Kansas University Center on Developmental Disabilities
- Andrés Gallegos, National Council on Disability

Moderator
Sandra Schneider, American College of Emergency Physicians

3:55–4:05 Closing Remarks

Panelists
Rick Gilfillan, former Director of the CMS Innovation Center

Appendix B

Statement of Task

A planning committee of the National Academies of Sciences, Engineering, and Medicine will plan a public workshop that will explore the challenges and opportunities related to building an optimal integrated care system for people with intellectual and developmental disabilities (IDD) (e.g., individuals with autism spectrum disorder). The workshop will feature invited presentations and discussions that will explore questions related to models of care, workforce, and financing and payment for care such as the following:

Models of Care
- What are illustrative examples of care models that deliver holistic, tailored (developmentally appropriate and patient-centered), and coordinated care?
- What factors limit the sustainability and/or adoption of these care models?

Workforce Issues
- What is known about the workforce that serves people with IDD?
- What are the facilitators and barriers to improving the competency and capacity of all clinicians to care for people with IDD, particularly for minority and poor populations?

Financing of and Payment for Care
- What key data/analytic gaps do payers and purchasers need addressed to design effective financing and payment approaches for IDD care?
- What policy or programmatic changes would be required to ensure appropriate levels of financing for IDD health care services, including support for clinical providers to coordinate with peers in other service domains?

The planning committee will plan and organize the workshop, identify speakers and discussants, and moderate discussions. A proceedings of the presentations and discussion at the workshop will be prepared by a designated rapporteur in accordance with institutional guidelines.

Appendix C

Biographical Sketches of the Speakers and Moderators

DAY ONE

Introductory Remarks

Kimberly Knackstedt, PH.D., M.Ed., is the director of disability policy for the Domestic Policy Council. She was the senior disability policy advisor for Senator Patty Murray on the Health, Education, Labor, and Pensions Committee in the U.S. Senate. Before that, she served as the disability policy advisor for Chairman Bobby Scott on the Committee on Education and Labor in the U.S. House of Representatives. She received her bachelor of education in special education and elementary education from Gonzaga University and master of education in special education and Ph.D. in special education and policy from the University of Kansas.

I. Elements and Competencies of an Integrated System of Care

Moderator: James M. Perrin, M.D., is professor of pediatrics at Harvard Medical School and the John C. Robinson Distinguished Chair in Pediatrics at the Massachusetts General Hospital. He was president (2014) of the American Academy of Pediatrics, chair of its Committee on Children with Disabilities, and president of the Ambulatory (Academic) Pediatric Association. He directed the Autism Intervention Research Network on Physical Health for 7 years and was founding editor of *Academic Pediatrics*. An elected member of the National Academy of Medicine, he has served on the boards of Family

Voices, the Frank Porter Graham Child Development Institute (University of North Carolina), and the Institute for Exceptional Care.

Edward Schor, M.D., is a pediatrician and an independent consultant providing advice on child health care systems and child health policy. Most recently, he served as senior vice president at the Lucile Packard Foundation for Children's Health, whose grantmaking focuses on health care system improvement for children with chronic and complex health conditions, where he initiated a variety of project defining standards for health care systems standards, care coordination, and family engagement. He has held senior positions with the Commonwealth Fund, where he worked to improve preventive child health care, Kaiser Family Foundation, where he promoted the adoption of functional health status measurement, and Iowa Department of Public Health, where he was medical director for Family and Community Health and director of the Center for Public Health Policy. He has written extensively on the family context of child health.

Lisa I. Iezzoni, M.D., M.Sc., is a professor of medicine, Harvard Medical School, and based at the Health Policy Research Center, Mongan Institute, Massachusetts General Hospital. Dr. Iezzoni has conducted numerous studies examining health care disparities for persons with disability. Her book *When Walking Fails* was published in 2003, and *More Than Ramps: A Guide to Improving Health Care Quality and Access for People with Disabilities*, coauthored with Bonnie O'Day, appeared in 2006. Representing Boston Center for Independent Living, she chaired the Medical Diagnostic Equipment Accessibility Standards Advisory Committee for the U.S. Access Board (2012–2013). Dr. Iezzoni is a member of the National Academy of Medicine.

Nanfi N. Lubogo, CCHW, is co-executive director for PATH CT, a statewide family support organization for families of children and youth with special health care needs/disabilities. She serves on various committees, councils, and boards both in CT and nationally. Her appointments include vice president of the Family Voices board of directors, co-lead of the Family Voices United to End Racism Against Children and Youth with Special Health Care Needs (CYSHCN) and Families project, American Academy of Pediatrics Council on Children with Disabilities EDI Workgroup, and National Emergency Medical Services for Children (EMSC) Family Advisory Network. Ms. Lubogo is a former council member of the National Emergency Medical Services Advisory Council, where she served as cochair of the Education and Preparedness committee. Ms. Lubogo is a Maternal and Child Health/Public Health Leadership Fellow and Partners in Policy Making Graduate.

II. Challenges in Workforce Strength and Preparedness

Moderator: Kara Ayers, Ph.D., is the associate director and an associate professor at the University of Cincinnati Center for Excellence in Developmental Disabilities (UCCEDD). She is director of the Center for Dignity in Healthcare for People with Disabilities and also a cofounder of the Disabled Parenting Project. Dr. Ayers' interests include disability identity/culture, health care equity, bioethics, community inclusion, and the use of media to teach, empower, and reduce stigma. She serves on multiple task forces and national and state coalitions related to improving outcomes for people with disabilities and infuses the mantra "Nothing about us without us" into all of her scholarly and community-based pursuits.

Matthew Holder, M.D., M.B.A., is recognized as an international leader in the emerging field of developmental medicine. Across the United States and around the world, his achievements in the development of clinical protocol, global health policy, and academic programming have improved the lives of tens of thousands of individuals with IDD. He is global medical advisor and chair of the Medical Advisory Committee for Special Olympics, International, CEO of Chyron and Advantage Medical Corp., and executive director and then president emeritus of the American Academy of Developmental Medicine and Dentistry.

Susan Havercamp's research contributions lie in three areas: building a health surveillance evidence base, developing and evaluating health promotion interventions, and improving health care for patients with disabilities. Recognizing that the U.S. health care system is ill prepared to meet these patients' needs, Dr. Havercamp partnered with people with disabilities and disability and health professionals to develop core competencies to guide training for health care professionals. She develops and implements disability training, helping to build a disability-competent health care workforce.

Amy Hewitt, Ph.D., has an extensive background in the IDD field. She has worked in various positions over the past 38 years to improve community inclusion and quality of life for children and adults with disabilities and their families. Her career began as a DSP, and she currently employs DSPs to support her brother-in-law. She is the director of the University of Minnesota's Institute on Community Integration and conducts research, evaluation, and demonstration projects about community services for children, youth, and adults with IDD and the DSP workforce. She has authored numerous journal articles, curriculum, and technical reports, including a book entitled *Staff Recruitment, Retention and Training*. Dr. Hewitt is on the editorial board of *Inclusion* and associate editor of *Intellectual and Developmental Disabilities*, both journals of the American Association on Intellectual and Developmental Disabilities (AAIDD). She is a past president of the Association of University Centers on Disability and AAIDD.

Spotlight Presentation

Maura Sullivan is the director of Operation House Call, a partnership between the Arc of Massachusetts and all major Massachusetts medical schools. This program teaches medical students and graduate nursing students the essential skills to enhance health care of persons with autism and other IDD. She is also the director of Government Affairs for the Arc; her work focuses on advocacy at the Massachusetts State House for people with disabilities. She is a national public speaker on health equity and a former LEND Fellow with an M.A. in public administration from Suffolk University. She is also the mother of three; her two sons have autism and mitochondrial disease.

III. Challenges in Financing and Payment

Moderator: Hoangmai (Mai) H. Pham is president of the Institute for Exceptional Care, a nonprofit dedicated to transforming health care for people with IDD. Dr. Pham is a general internist and national health policy leader. She was vice president at Anthem, responsible for value-based care initiatives. Prior to Anthem, Dr. Pham served as chief innovation officer at the CMMI, where she was a founding official and the architect of foundational programs on accountable care organizations and primary care. Dr. Pham has published extensively on provider payment policy and its intersection with health disparities, quality performance, provider behavior, and market trends. She serves on numerous advisory bodies, including for the National Academy of Medicine, National Advisory Council for the Agency on Healthcare Research and Quality, and Maryland Primary Care Program. Dr. Pham earned her A.B. from Harvard University, her M.D. from Temple University, and her M.P.H. from Johns Hopkins University, where she was also a Robert Wood Johnson Clinical Scholar.

Michael Monson is president and CEO of Altarum, a nonprofit health care consulting and research organization committed to improving the health of individuals with fewer financial resources and populations disenfranchised by the health care system. He is leading the next stage of Altarum's growth, focused on transforming service delivery, advancing public health, integrating public health and service delivery, and scaling health infrastructure. Most recently, he was CEO of Social Health Bridge at Centene Corporation and senior vice president of Medicaid and Complex Care, where he had national product responsibility for Centene's Medicaid and Complex Care product lines, which included TANF, CHIP, foster care, Medicaid expansion, LTSS, ABD, and dual eligibles. He developed Centene's strategy to address the social determinants of health and led its Center for Health Transformation, a collaboration with academic researchers that improved quality of care across its 12.5 million members in 30 states. He began his work in health care leading strategy and innovation at the Visiting Nurse Service of New York, a safety net organization that was also the nation's largest home-based health care company. He was chief administrative officer at Village Care of New York, an integrated health system, where he ran multiple residential facilities and multiple corporate functions.

Ari Ne'eman is a Ph.D. candidate in health policy at Harvard University, senior research associate at the Harvard Law School Project on Disability, and visiting scholar at the Lurie Institute for Disability Policy. He was executive director of the Autistic Self Advocacy Network (2006–2016) and one of President Obama's appointees to the NCD (2010–2015). He is working on a book on the history of American disability advocacy for Simon & Schuster.

Cheryl Powell is a health care executive with over two decades of experience in Medicaid, Medicare, and private health insurance policy, financing, and operations. She works with national leaders to transform our health care system to be more person driven through financing, payment incentive design, and delivery system reform. She has held a variety of leadership roles at CMS, IBM Watson Health, and MITRE (the Health Federally Funded Research and Development Center). In these roles, she has led major national reform and policy initiatives, including person-driven care and alignment of financial incentives to enhance care value and outcomes. She has an M.A. in public policy from the Kennedy School of Government at Harvard University and a B.A. from the University of Virginia.

DAY TWO

IV. Innovative Models of Care & Care Coordination

Moderator: Elizabeth Mahar is the director of Family & Sibling Initiatives at the Arc, National. She has nearly 20 years of experience in government affairs, public relations, and nonprofit sectors. Ms. Mahar has created partnerships for government and corporate clients with their target audiences to achieve measurable campaign results. She has significant experience in account management, local and national partnership development, event planning and execution, multicultural outreach, bilingual communications, marketing and strategy development, and implementation, writing, and editing.

Clarissa Kripke is clinical professor of Family and Community Medicine and Director of Developmental Primary Care at the University of California San Francisco. She provides primary medical care to some of the San Francisco Bay Area's most medically fragile and behaviorally complex clients with developmental disabilities. She ran a multidisciplinary, mobile consult and assessment service in Northern California for people who were moving from institutions or at risk of institutionalization. She trains health professionals how to apply social model and neurodiversity models of disability to the practice of medicine.

Patricia Aguayo, M.D, M.P.H., is medical director of the HOME program and Autism Spectrum Disorder Clinic. She graduated from the Universidad Anahuac Medical School in Mexico City. Dr. Aguayo completed a psychiatry residency at New York Medical College and a child and adolescent psychiatry fellowship at the Yale Child Study Center. She holds an M.P.H. from the University of Arizona. She is the parent of a young adult with autism spectrum disorder (ASD) and has worked in the field of ASD for most of her career.

Lauren Easton served as the behavioral health leader for CCA. Over the years and in various roles, she has been largely responsible for developing CCA's behavioral health integration across its care models and creating a responsive network and many innovative programs. She embraced the integration of behavioral health and medical care long before it became "trendy." She has made behavioral health integration a hallmark of program development throughout her professional life. She is responsible for the oversight of CCA's behavioral health services, delivered through its network of behavioral health providers and specialists to its 17,000+ members. She oversees the development and expansion of the One Care program, paying particular attention to the significant mental health needs of this population. She provides consultation, education, and support to clinicians and others in a provider network regarding behavioral health/substance abuse treatment and management and ensures that the organization can appropriately and effectively support the needs of enrollees with mental illness and other behavioral health needs. She actively collaborates with state agencies and legislators to support the development of innovative behavioral health services and programs throughout the state.

Spotlight Presentation

Vijay Ravindran is the cofounder and CEO of Floreo, a start-up building virtual reality autism therapy. He was the chief digital officer of a major media company, chief executive of a news start-up, and cofounder of a political technology company that was active in the 2008 presidential campaign. He started his career as a software engineer and was at Amazon (1998–2005) in a variety of technology roles, including technology director. In 2005, he joined former White House Deputy Chief of Staff Harold Ickes to launch the political technology start-up Catalist. As its founding chief technology officer, he led all the technology aspects of developing its software and data products. During the 2008 election cycle, Catalist clients included the Obama for America and Hillary Clinton presidential campaigns. He graduated from the University of Virginia with a B.S. in systems engineering.

V. Innovations in Workforce Solutions: Role of General Health Care Providers

Moderator: Susan Hingle is an internal medicine specialist and a professor of medicine who serves as associate dean for Human and Organizational Potential and director of Faculty Development at Southern Illinois University School of Medicine. She is active in organized medicine, having served as chair of the American College of Physicians board of regents and board of governors. She is on the American Medical Women's Association board of directors and the American Medical Association's Women Physician Section Governing Council. She has a son who is on the autism spectrum and has suffered from intolerance, inflexibility, and lack of compassion and understanding. Dr. Hingle strongly believes that we must focus on equity and inclusion broadly to be able to reach our full potential as individuals, organizations, and professions. She earned a B.A. from Miami University and an M.D. from Rush University Medical College and completed an internal medicine residency at Georgetown University.

Kristin Sohl, M.D., FAAP, is a professor of clinical child health at the University of Missouri and founder and executive director of ECHO Autism, a global program partnering with clinicians and professionals to increase access to autism best practices. As a pediatrician with extensive experience in medical diagnosis, evaluation, and longitudinal support of people with autism and other developmental/behavioral disorders, she is a tireless advocate for children's health, particularly related to changing systems to improve access to equitable care in rural and underserved locations. She is the president of the American Academy of Pediatrics, Missouri Chapter and the chair of the American Academy of Pediatrics, Autism Subcommittee within the Council on Children with Disabilities. She completed medical school and pediatric residency at the University of Missouri.

Lisa Howley, Ph.D., is senior director for the AAMC Transformation of Medical Education and adjunct associate professor at University of North Carolina Chapel Hill School of Medicine. She is an educational psychologist who has spent over 25 years in the field of medical education supporting learners and faculty, conducting research, and developing curricula. She joined the AAMC in 2016 to advance the continuum of medical education and support experiential learning and curricular transformation across its member institutions and their clinical partners. Before that, she spent 8 years as the associate Designated Institutional Official and Assistant Vice President of Medical Education and Physician Development for Carolinas HealthCare System in North Carolina, one of the largest independent academic medical centers in the United States, where she led a number of medical education initiatives across the professional development continuum, including graduate medical education accreditation and physician leadership development. She began her medical education career at the University of Virginia School of Medicine, where she designed and integrated clinical skills performance assessments and experiential learning activities across the medical curricula. She received her B.A. in psychology from the University of Central Florida and both her M.A. and Ph.D. in educational psychology from the University of Virginia.

Sarah Ailey, Ph.D., RN, FAAN, is a professor of nursing at Rush University in Chicago, Illinois. She is the principal investigator for the Partnering to Transform Health Outcomes with Persons with Intellectual and Developmental Disabilities Program (path-pwidd.org), funded through a 5-year grant from the Administration for Community Living. She is the president of the Alliance for Disability in Health Care Education (ADHCE.org).

VI. Innovations in Financing and Payment

Moderator: Hoangmai (Mai) H. Pham is president of the Institute for Exceptional Care, a nonprofit dedicated to transforming health care for people with IDD. Dr. Pham is a general internist and national health policy leader. She was vice president at Anthem, responsible for value-based care initiatives. Before that, Dr. Pham served as chief innovation officer at the CMMI, where she was a founding official, and the architect of foundational programs on accountable care organizations and primary care. Dr. Pham has published extensively on provider payment policy and its intersection with health disparities, quality performance, provider behavior, and market trends. She serves on numerous advisory bodies, including for the National Academy of Medicine, National Advisory Council for the Agency on Healthcare Research and Quality, and Maryland Primary Care Program. Dr. Pham earned her A.B. from Harvard University, her M.D. from Temple University, and her M.P.H.

from Johns Hopkins University, where she was also a Robert Wood Johnson Clinical Scholar.

Brede Eschliman is director of Medicare at Aurrera Health Group. Before that, she was a program examiner in the Medicare Branch at the Office of Management and Budget, where she reviewed, revised, and recommended clearance or nonconcurrence of proposed Medicare regulations and CMMI alternative payment models. She also spent several years working at CMMI, where she led model teams in designing, implementing, and improving alternative payment models, and as the director of operations at a community health center, where she oversaw revenue cycle activities, supervised practice managers and front desk staff, and conducted rapid-cycle process improvement to improve patient access and price transparency.

Sarah Hudson Scholle, D.P.H., Johns Hopkins University, is vice president of Research and Analysis at the NCQA. Dr. Scholle is an expert in health services and quality measurement in multiple settings and has a demonstrated record of moving innovative concepts into implementation through NCQA's programs and Healthcare Effectiveness Data and Information Set. Dr. Scholle's expertise ranges from equity and person-centered care to delivery system improvement. Her work on equity has addressed disparities in care, methods for summarizing and incentivizing health equity, and approaches for improving data. She has conducted numerous projects to advance the use of patient-reported outcomes in clinical care and quality measurement, including a novel approach to personalized goal setting.

Stephanie Rasmussen is the vice president of Long-Term Supports & Services for Sunflower Health Plan in Kansas. She has over 32 years of experience in LTSS, including providing direct services for persons with IDD, administration of an IDD provider association, and consultation in three states on the development of services for persons with IDD being placed out of closing state institutional settings. She has been with Sunflower Health, a managed long-term supports and services plan owned by Centene Corporation, for 9 years.

DAY THREE

VII. A New Vision for Models of Care

Moderator: Kara Ayers, Ph.D., is the associate director and an associate professor at the UCCEDD. She is director of the Center for Dignity in Healthcare for People with Disabilities and also a cofounder of the Disabled Parenting Project. Dr. Ayers' interests include disability identity/culture, health care equity, bioethics, community inclusion, and the use of media to teach, empower, and reduce stigma. She serves on multiple task forces and national and state coalitions related to improving outcomes for people with disabilities and infuses the mantra "Nothing about us without us" into all of her scholarly and community-based pursuits.

Moderator: Alicia Theresa Francesca Bazzano, Ph.D., is the chief health officer of Special Olympics. Dr. Bazzano provides strategic oversight of health activities around the world to ensure public funding, policies, medical training programs, and health service delivery are inclusive of people with intellectual disabilities. She is a pediatrician and public health executive who has dedicated her career to improving the health of people with intellectual disabilities. Prior to joining Special Olympics in 2019, she served as senior medical director for Health Policy at Acumen and chief physician at the Westside Regional Center in Los Angeles, which serves individuals with IDD. Dr. Bazzano was also deeply involved in founding the Achievable Health Center, a first-of-its-kind federally qualified health center dedicated to developmental disabilities, and served as founding cochief medical officer. Dr. Bazzano completed medical school and pediatric residency at UCLA and was a UCLA Clinical Scholar, selected by the Robert Wood Johnson Foundation. She also completed her M.P.H. and Ph.D. in the Department of Health Policy and Management at UCLA.

John A. Kitzhaber, M.D., graduated from University of Oregon Medical School and practiced emergency medicine in Roseburg, Oregon. He served in the Oregon House and State Senate and as Oregon's longest-serving governor (1995–2003 and 2011–2015). He authored the Oregon Health Plan in 1989, which built a defined benefit based on a prioritized list of health service, and is a chief architect of Oregon's coordinated care organizations, which now provide care to over a million Oregonians within a global budget indexed to a sustainable growth rate, while meeting quality and outcome metrics. In 2013, *Modern Healthcare Magazine* ranked him #2 on the list of the "100 Most Influential People in Health Care" and #1 on the list of the "50 Most Influential Physician Executives." He is a writer, speaker and private consultant on health policy and politics, and chair of health policy at the Foundation for Medical Excellence.

Sharon Lewis is a nationally lauded expert in disability policy spanning HCBS, education, employment, independent living supports, and person-centered services. She is a principal at Health Management Associates and works with federal partners, states, providers, and consumer advocates to advance opportunities for people with disabilities to fully participate in all aspects of community, across the life-span. Ms. Lewis is a collaborator and

APPENDIX C   111

consensus builder with a natural ability to put policy into practical perspective. She has served in presidentially appointed leadership roles at the U.S. Department of HHS, including principal deputy administrator of the Administration for Community Living, senior disability policy advisor to the HHS Secretary, and commissioner of the Administration on Intellectual and Developmental Disabilities.

Charlene Wong, M.D., MSHP, is an assistant professor of pediatrics and public policy at Duke University and the Duke-Margolis Center for Health Policy. She is the executive director of the North Carolina Integrated Care for Kids model. As a pediatrician and health services researcher, she researches health care transformation and health-related behavior change, leveraging principles from behavioral economics and employing a person-centered approach to research and policy. She is a leader in value-based payment models for child and family health. She serves as the program director for Health Behaviors and Needs Research in the Duke Children's Health & Discovery Initiative and associate program director for the National Clinician Scholars Program at Duke. Her research training includes fellowships at CDC and in the Robert Wood Johnson Foundation Clinical Scholars Program.

Spotlight Presentation

Maulik M. Trivedi is a board-certified emergency medicine physician in practice for over 20 years and was the chair or associate chair of several EDs. He continues to practice in the NYC area. He is a founding partner of StationMD and has been instrumental in helping it achieve its mission of improving the quality of care for the population with IDD. He is a recognized national speaker and thought leader on using technology and telehealth solutions to positively impact medical care and foster independence. He and his family live in midtown Manhattan.

VIII. Technical and Policy Opportunities in Financing and Payment

Moderator: Julia Bascom serves as executive director at the Autistic Self Advocacy Network (ASAN). ASAN was created to serve as a national grassroots disability rights organization for the autistic community, advocating for systems change and ensuring that the voices of autistic people are heard in policy debates and the halls of power. ASAN believes that the goal of autism advocacy should be a world in which autistic people enjoy equal access, rights, and opportunities. ASAN focuses substantial attention on health care policy and policy regarding HCBS. She also serves on the advisory board of Felicity

House, Anthem's National Advisory Board, and the boards of the Consortium for Citizens with Disabilities, the Institute for Exceptional Care, and Allies For Independence.

Alyna Chien is a physician researcher based at Harvard Medical School and Boston Children's Hospital and focused on the relationship between incentives and disparities. After providing most of the available empirical information on the effectiveness of value-based purchasing and care quality for children, she created the Children with Disabilities Algorithm and received an R01 from the Eunice Kennedy Shriver National Institute of Child Health and Human Development to examine health care transitions for adolescents and young adults with IDD. Dr. Chien's national committee service has included the Patient Centered Outcome Research Institute (Disparities), National Quality Forum (Risk Adjustment), CMMI (Next Generation Accountable Care Organizations), and National Academies of Medicine (Value Incentives and System Innovation Collaborative). However, at the beginning and end of each day, she is the proud aunt, godmother, and sister-in-law to family members with IDD.

Colleen Kidney is a policy associate at Human Services Research Institute, where she consults with jurisdictions undertaking systems redesign initiatives for their HCBS waiver programs. She specializes in developing individual budget methodologies using assessment of support needs. Her work emphasizes data-driven and stakeholder-engaged approaches to promoting equity and self-determination in individuals with IDD. Dr. Kidney received her Ph.D. in applied community psychology from Portland State University and resides in Portland, Oregon.

Joan Alker is the executive director and cofounder of the Center for Children and Families and a research professor at the Georgetown University McCourt School of Public Policy. She is a nationally recognized expert on Medicaid and CHIP and the lead author of an annual report on children's health care coverage trends. Other recent work areas include "Children's Health Insurance Coverage: Progress, Problems and Beyond" Health Affairs 2020, a series of reports looking at Medicaid's role in rural areas, and a great deal of work on Section 1115 waivers. She holds an M.Phil. in politics from St. Antony's College, Oxford University, and a B.A. with honors in political science from Bryn Mawr College.

Joshua M. Sharfstein is professor of the Practice in Health Policy and Management at the Johns Hopkins Bloomberg School of Public Health, where he also serves as vice dean for Public Health Practice and Community Engagement and as director of the Bloomberg American Health Initiative. He is a former health commissioner of Baltimore, principal deputy commissioner of the U.S. Food and Drug Administration, and health secretary of Maryland. Dr. Sharfstein teaches a class called "Crisis and Response in Public Health Policy and Practice" and authored *Public Health Crisis Survival Guide: Leadership and Management in Trying Times* (2018) and coauthored *The Opioid Epidemic: What Everyone Needs to Know* (2019).

IX. SCALING WORKFORCE SOLUTIONS

Moderator: Sandra Schneider, M.D., FACEP, is the senior vice president for Clinical Affairs at the American College of Emergency Physicians and adjunct professor of emergency medicine at the University of Pittsburgh. She was the founding chair of the Department of Emergency Medicine at the University of Rochester. She is a former president of the American College of Emergency Physicians, Society for Academic Emergency Medicine, and Association of Academic Chairs of Emergency Medicine. She is the author of over 100 peer-reviewed publications and over 50 textbook chapters.

Helen Burstin, M.D., M.P.H., MACP, is the CEO of the Council of Medical Specialty Societies, a coalition of 47 specialty societies representing more than 800,000 physicians. Dr. Burstin was scientific officer of the National Quality Forum. She serves on the boards of AcademyHealth and the Society to Improve Diagnosis in Medicine. Dr. Burstin is the author of more than 100 articles and book chapters on quality, safety, equity, and measurement. She is a clinical professor of medicine at George Washington University School of Medicine and Health Sciences. Her recent awards include the Alpha Omega Alpha Medical Voluntary Attending Award from the George Washington School of Medicine and Mastership from the American College of Physicians.

Karrie A. Shogren, Ph.D., is director of the Center on Developmental Disabilities (a University Center for Excellence in Developmental Disabilities), senior scientist at the Schiefelbusch Life Span Institute, and professor in the Department of Special Education, all at the University of Kansas. Dr. Shogren's research focuses on assessment and intervention in self-determination and supported decision making for people with disabilities. She has led multiple grant-funded projects, including assessment validation and efficacy trials of self-determination interventions in school and community contexts. Dr. Shogren has published over 200 articles in peer-reviewed journals, authored or coauthored 10 books, and is the lead author of the Self-Determination Inventory (www.self-determination.org), a recently validated assessment of self-determination and the Supported Decision-Making Inventory System, the first assessment of the supports needed to involve people with IDD in decisions about their lives.

Andrés J. Gallegos, Esq., is the chair of the NCD, appointed to that position by President Biden on the afternoon of his inauguration. NCD is an independent federal agency mandated to advise the president, administration, Congress, and federal agencies on all policy matters affecting people with disabilities in the United States and its territories. He is also a disability rights and health care law attorney in Chicago, Illinois, with Robbins, Salomon & Patt, where he founded and directs the national disability rights practice. He is a person with a disability, having sustained a spinal cord injury resulting in quadriplegia 25 years ago.

CLOSING REMARKS

Richard J. "Rick" Gilfillan is president and CEO of Trinity Health, the $15.9 billion Catholic health system that serves communities in 22 states with 92 hospitals, 120 continuing care locations, and home health and hospice facilities that provide more than 2.5 million home health and hospice visits annually. For more than 30 years, he has built successful organizations in the for-profit and not-for-profit sectors to deliver better outcomes for people and communities. As the first director of the CMMI, he launched it in 2010 and worked quickly with payers and providers to develop innovative models for improving patient care and reducing costs.

Before that, he was president and CEO of Geisinger Health Plan and executive vice president of insurance operations for Geisinger Health System, a large integrated health system in Pennsylvania. He was the senior vice president for national network management at Coventry Health Care. He also held earlier executive positions at Independence Blue Cross.

He began his career as a family medicine physician and later became a medical director and a chief medical officer. He earned his undergraduate and medical degrees from Georgetown University and an M.B.A. from the Wharton School of the University of Pennsylvania.